$$\boxed{\text{NAS}}$$

ALTSCHUL'S PSYCHIATRIC AND MENTAL HEALTH NURSING

Seventh Edition

Margaret McGovern

MSc(Edin), BA(Lond), RGN, RMN, RCNT, RNT, HVDip

Nurse Teacher,
Lothian College of Health Studies

Sarah Whitcher

MA(Edin), RGN, RMN, CPN(Cert), CPNT

Quality Co-ordinator,
Mental Health Services,
Addenbrookes NHS Trust

Baillière Tindall
London   Philadelphia   Toronto   Sydney   Tokyo

Baillière Tindall   24–28 Oval Road
W. B. Saunders   London NW1 7DX

The Curtis Center
Independence Square West
Philadelphia, PA 19106–3399, USA

Harcourt Brace & Company
55 Horner Avenue
Toronto, Ontario, M8Z 4X6, Canada

Harcourt Brace & Company, Australia
30–52 Smidmore Street
Marrickville
NSW 2204, Australia

Harcourt Brace & Company, Japan
Ichibancho Central Building
22–1 Ichibancho
Chiyoda-ku, Tokyo 102, Japan

First published 1957
Seventh edition 1994
German translation, third edition, 1972 (Urban & Schwarzenberg,
Munich)
Spanish translation, fifth edition, 1977 (CECSA, Mexico)
Portuguese translation, fifth edition, 1977 (Publicações Europa-
América, Mem-Martins, Sintra)
Dutch translation, fifth edition, 1979 (Stafleu, Alphen)
Fifth ELBS edition 1979
Sixth edition 1985

This book is printed on acid-free paper

A catalogue record for this book is available from the British Library

ISBN 0–7020–1412–5

Typeset by Phoenix Photosetting, Chatham
Printed and bound in Great Britain by
Mackays of Chatham PLC, Chatham, Kent

Contents

Foreword

In the forty years since I started to prepare the first edition of this book, many colleagues have been contributing knowledge and experience. In particular my co-authors, first Ruth Simpson and latterly Margaret McGovern, have been keeping me up-to-date and I am greatly indebted to them.

My continuing involvement, in various ways, with people suffering from mental disorder, makes me believe that little has changed in the nature of psychiatric illness or the principles on which successful treatment is based. What has changed beyond recognition is the setting in which treatment nowadays takes place and the speed with which improvement or recovery are expected to occur.

I have not been able to keep up with the changes in nursing education and nursing practice and have not been involved in this revision. I am delighted that Sarah Whitcher's expertise in community psychiatric nursing and her management experience have been made available to Margaret McGovern as her co-author.

When I wrote the first edition of the book, student psychiatric nurses obtained their entire training within mental hospitals, where their prolonged experience in different types of wards and departments qualified them to provide patients with lasting relationships and continuity of care. 'Short stay' then, was measured in months of inpatient treatment, 'long stay' in years. Students learned to use the hospital environment and their own personality in such a way that patients were able to make maximal use of the therapeutic potential available. Of course there were dangers associated with this method of care: that patients and staff would become institutionalized;

that in their zeal to provide good custodial care, staff might overlook opportunities to promote the patients' independence; that after long periods of hospitalization patients and their relatives might have difficulties in readjusting to the demands of the community; and that, for nurses, training for hospital work might be counter-productive in the community, which for many nurses was to become the preferred or the only available career path. Previous editions of this book dealt in some detail with methods of preventing 'institutional neurosis', of re-motivating, re-educating and rehabilitating patients in preparation for discharge. The need for post-registration training in community nursing was taken for granted. This new edition shows clearly that the same principles apply wherever nurses and patients meet and that the dangers need not arise with the current, much less leisurely approach to psychiatric nursing.

All students of nursing now have the opportunity of meeting people suffering from mental disorder in the community as well as in hospital. They no longer need to unlearn hospital practice before being able to meet the patients' needs at home. During the branch programme, longer allocation to psychiatric wards or with community psychiatric nurses will provide the opportunity to develop therapeutic relationships. Even by the end of the course the newly qualified mental health nurses may feel that not enough has been learnt about the complexity of human problems. They may still feel insecure in the management of difficult situations.

I am confident that this book will be a useful companion to the student in the wide and varied exposure to patients. The positive approach which the authors convey will ensure that the newly qualified mental health nurse rapidly becomes a knowledgeable expert and skilled practitioner.

ANNIE ALTSCHUL

Preface

An important feature of this new edition is the equal emphasis given to the care of the person with mental health problems in the community; previous editions have been almost exclusively concerned with the care of the person in hospital. This radical departure gives expression to the fact that the mental health needs of the overwhelming majority of people are met outside hospital and reflects the trend—accelerated significantly in recent years—towards a more community-based pattern of psychiatric services. It will be noted therefore that in order to avoid repetition, detailed descriptions of care which is similar irrespective of the setting in which it occurs may be given either from the community psychiatric nurse's perspective or, as in the rehabilitation of a long-stay resident, from that of the hospital-based nurse.

A further innovation in this edition is the use of quotations from those who have had personal experience of psychiatric help. It is our view that these are invaluable for the psychiatric and mental health nurse to achieve success as an empathetic practitioner.

The last but by no means the least significant change is that of the principal author of previous editions of *Psychiatric Nursing*. The current authors, former students of Annie Altschul, each owe her an inestimable debt and hope that much of her teaching is in evidence throughout the pages of this text.

No attempt has been made in this introductory text to give a comprehensive account of all aspects of mental health and psychiatric nursing care. Omissions such as the specialist areas of child and adolescent nursing care, eating disorders and substance abuse can be repaired by

referring to the many excellent texts by expert nurse practitioners which are currently available. Similarly Chapter
10 (Caring for the Elderly Person who is Confused) does
not include a detailed description of the physical needs of
the elderly person in hospital; these are well covered in
standard texts devoted entirely to this highly skilled and
challenging field of nursing practice.

For reasons of readability only, the person in need of
care is usually referred to throughout this book in the
male gender and the nurse in the female. In view of the
ongoing debate regarding the 'name' given to the person
who is receiving care, we have after careful consideration
decided that we will use that term which appears most
appropriate in the context. Therefore, the terms 'patient',
'resident', 'client' and 'person' are used interchangeably,
though the more frequent use of 'person' reflects our
preference.

MARGARET MCGOVERN
SARAH WHITCHER

SECTION I: GENERAL INTRODUCTION

Chapter 1
Mental Health and Mental Illness

Psychiatric and mental health nursing is concerned with:

- the promotion of mental health;
- the prevention of mental ill-health; and
- the nursing care of people who suffer from mental health problems.

Thus the introductory part of the book begins with a general discussion of the concept of mental health, followed by a brief historical overview of psychiatric care and treatment in the past and an account of how society's attitudes towards mental illness have changed over time. Chapter 2 closes with an overview of current issues in mental health.

Chapter 3—Section II of this book—is largely devoted to a discussion of the organization of care in the community which has as its principal aim the promotion of mental health and the prevention of mental ill-health. A description of some of the innovations in the practice of nursing in the community and in an inpatient setting follows in Chapter 4.

The nursing care of people with mental health needs takes up all of the chapters in Section III of the book. Emphasis is firmly placed on a holistic approach to nursing care, and focuses on the individual's emotional responses and behavioural reactions in preference to the particular diagnostic label used by other members of the multidisciplinary team.

Section IV includes specific therapeutic interventions which may be required to supplement or complement those already discussed and contains a description of psychological therapies and of the physical treatment, electroconvulsive therapy (ECT).

The text closes with a discussion of the future challenges to be faced in the field of mental health and highlights some of the possible implications of the new and projected changes in legislation in mental health care.

Appendix A, 'Classification and Description of some Psychiatric Disorders', acknowledges that nurses need to know something of the disorders they hope to help prevent and to treat. The reader is referred to this appendix when a fuller description of the clinical features of specific disorders may prove helpful. Equally the nurse should be conversant with the legal rights of a person who may be compulsorily detained in hospital. Appendix B gives a description of these rights and also some relevant details of current legislation. The remainder of the appendices contain information about some of the drugs in common use in psychiatric practice, examples of scales used when caring for the person who is anxious, and finally some useful addresses of agencies—mainly voluntary—offering help to those with mental health problems.

This chapter will look briefly at the concept of mental health, including a brief discussion of what may be regarded as normality and the effects of social change on mental health.

NORMALITY AND MENTAL HEALTH

Many textbooks of medicine and nursing begin with a description of the normal and proceed to describe the abnormal conditions which arise in ill-health. Originally, however, knowledge of what is normal and healthy in body and mind was nearly always gained by studying what was abnormal and diseased. Knowledge of the normal functioning of endocrine glands, for example, was discovered as a result of studying abnormalities associated with over- or under-production of hormones. Normal functioning of the brain becomes clearer as more and more is known about people suffering from brain lesions. The study of mental health, which has been defined by World Health Organization as 'the full and harmonious functioning of the whole personality', may also be enlightened by reference to mental disorder. Nurses in seeking to promote mental health need to know what to regard as healthy and what signs to interpret as evidence of mental ill-health. As they become acquainted with abnormal behaviour they will develop a clear idea of the standards by which they can judge the behaviour of those in their care, and of what to regard as normal.

THE DEFINITION OF NORMALITY

What is meant by normality? What does normal life entail? It is often said that we are all 'a bit abnormal'. Is this true or is it obvious nonsense? Is it any easier if the word 'normal' is replaced by 'healthy', or is it normal to be a little unhealthy?

The difficulty which arises in answering these questions

lies in the fact that the word 'normal' is used in more than one sense. It is sometimes employed for 'average' or 'most usual'. By 'normal height' is usually meant 'within certain limits around the average'. But the word 'normal' is not used in this sense when health is being discussed. For instance, it may be found that by a certain age many people have lost their teeth and are wearing dentures, but it is not therefore 'normal' to wear dentures by the age of, say, 65.

It is often preferred to consider 'normal' as being 'ideal' or 'best possible'. An individual would be called 'normal' in respect of physical health if his or her organs were functioning in the ideal manner, and 'ill-health' or 'abnormality' are the terms that would be used if there were any serious deviation from the optimal function.

Any particular characteristic or clinical symptom may thus be abnormal when judged by absolute standards, but normal when judged by population standards, or vice versa. Outstandingly high intelligence, for example, may approach normality in the sense of 'optimal', but it represents considerable deviation from the 'norm' by population standards.

Deviation from the population norm is not always morbid, as the example of exceptionally high intelligence shows. In old age it may be that a person formerly of outstandingly high intelligence declines to a level approaching the norm for the population as a whole. He or she then suffers from a disorder characterized by deviation of intelligence from a personal norm.

HOW ABOUT MENTAL HEALTH?

Here it is difficult to define the ideal without reference to society. It could be said that a person is *healthy* if they manage to deal with the demands made upon them by society in a manner which is ideal both for society and for themselves. They are *unhealthy* to the degree that they have failed in their adjustment, to the detriment either of society or of themselves. No definition is, however, entirely satisfactory. There are those who regard society as sick, perceiving those who deviate from the norms of society as healthy. To equate mental health with adjustment to society also gives rise to the impression that psychiatrists and psychiatric nurses are committed to maintaining the status quo and preventing social change.

SOCIAL CHANGE AND MENTAL HEALTH

Social change, however, cannot be prevented: it is an inevitable and necessary feature of our industrial society. Chapter 2 will survey some of the ways in which there have been important positive changes in society's attitudes towards people with mental health problems over the years; though not all social change is wholly beneficial to everyone. For example, the decline in the extended family has meant a loss of social contacts for a number of elderly people, and changes in the status, role and rights of women have coincided with a considerable increase in mothers struggling to bring up young children on their own. Brown and Harris (1978) found that socially and emotionally isolated mothers who—among other factors—were precluded from taking up outside employment by the presence of young children showed a vulnerability to mental illness. Further examples of some of the stressful effects of social change on a person's mental health will be outlined in later chapters.

FURTHER READING

Muijen M & Brooking JI (1989) *Mental Health*. In: White A (ed.)
  Health in the Inner City. Oxford: Heinemann.

REFERENCE

Brown G & Harris T (1978) *Social Origins of Depression: a Study of
  Psychiatric Disorder in Women*. London: Tavistock.

Chapter 2
The Psychiatrically Ill and Society: A Historical Review of Care and Treatment

INTRODUCTION

This chapter traces the extent to which society has effected change in both the attitude towards and treatment of mental illness. The enlightened opinion and courage of one or two doctors enabled a more humane approach to the treatment and management of people with mental illness. This eventually led to legislation to protect the rights of people suffering from a mental illness and to a recognition of the need to protect society from the unfortunate effects of the behaviour of some people suffering from a mental illness. This enlightened approach led to an increased interest in researching the cause and treatment of mental illness and in changing from custodial management to care in the community.

HISTORICAL REVIEW

Until the end of the last century, with isolated exceptions, those who suffered from mental disorder were ignored or ridiculed unless they were obviously dangerous to the community. Those who were thought to be dangerous were, at various periods, executed, ill-treated or imprisoned. They were considered as being totally different from other human beings, chained and kept under physical restraint, physically and mentally tortured in order to render them manageable.

Pinel in France (1745–1826), and Tuke in York (1732–1822), proclaimed that the insane person was human, and would respond to kindness. Pinel, watched by a frightened and disbelieving audience, removed the chains and convinced his followers that the time was ripe for humane treatment of the insane. Education was required, both of those who were responsible for the care of the insane, and of society as a whole, before some of the fear of the insane person was lost and sufficient sympathy and interest acquired to abandon restraint. In 1889 the first course of instruction was given to attendants of the insane in Britain.

As public opinion changed, so people became less disposed to hide their affliction, and it became clear how large was the number of people who would benefit by humane care. Lunatic asylums were built where many thousands were cared for, often placed there by relatives and a society unable or unwilling to understand and cope with the behaviour presented and only too ready to allow others to take the responsibility of providing that care.

Not until the end of the nineteenth century was the public conscience sufficiently aroused in England to accept, by Act of Parliament, official responsibility for the care of the insane, to delegate this duty to local authorities, and at the same time to admit that people of unsound mind required the protection of the law from those who might be sufficiently unscrupulous to take advantage of their afflictions.

The Lunacy Act of 1890 clearly laid down the circumstances in which society had the right to protect itself from those who might cause damage as a result of mental disorder. It defined the responsibility of the local authority to provide care and protection, free of charge, for those who were certified to be in need of them, and it laid down in detail the extent to which a person deprived of his liberty by virtue of certification was entitled to protection and to the safeguard of many of the rights of citizenship.

As time passed, many of the safeguards against wrongful certification, exploitation and ill-treatment appeared no longer to be necessary. Better staff were employed in mental hospitals, and public opinion had moved towards sympathy and understanding.

While wrongful certification became an unlikely occurrence, fear of mental illness and the stigma associated with it prevented maintenance of interest in the patient after certification. Feelings of fear, shame and guilt caused relatives to delay certification as long as possible but, once this had become necessary, quickly to forget the patient. The geographical situation of many asylums made visiting difficult, and there was a tendency to think of admission to an asylum as final. Many asylums, with their beautiful grounds, became self-contained communities, a refuge for patients from the harsh world outside.

CHANGING ATTITUDES TO PSYCHIATRIC DISORDERS

While public opinion gradually moved to an acceptance of responsibility for the humane care of the mentally disturbed, expert opinion approached the recognition of mental disorder as an illness requiring medical and nursing care. Medical interest was devoted to careful description of abnormal behaviour in an attempt to classify and diagnose it, and to prescribe treatment. Psychiatric nurses were needed in place of attendants for the insane. The new function of the nurse consisted of accurate recording of signs and symptoms, and in helping to detect early manifestations of psychiatric disorder with a view to treatment and prevention.

Fear of certification, however, militated against early treatment of psychiatric disorder, and a new method for the admission of patients became necessary. In 1930 the Mental Treatment Act made it possible to receive treatment in a mental hospital as a voluntary or temporary patient, without legal formalities, and yet retain the protection granted to certified patients. The Mental Treatment Act was preceded by a similar Act in Scotland, and in England by a special Act of Parliament granting the London County Council permission to treat voluntary patients at the Maudsley Hospital.

To emphasize the recognition of psychiatric disorder as illness the name 'asylum' was changed to 'mental hospital', the word 'patient' substituted for 'lunatic', and 'nurse' for 'attendant'.

Over time, many people became aware that the legislation relating to mental disorder was still unnecessarily complex and restrictive and began to campaign for changes in the legislation and in the treatment of people with mental health disorders. A Royal Commission was set up in 1954 to enquire into the way the law was operating and to make recommendations for change. As a result of it, the Mental Health Act was passed in 1959 and the Mental Health (Scotland) Act in 1960. They came into operation in 1961.

The essence of the Acts was reflected in the title. *Mental health* rather than disease was the subject of the Acts. All previous legislation relating to mental illness and to mental deficiency became obsolete and the aim of these Acts was to abolish many of the distinctions between the way people suffering from physical and mental disorder were treated.

The Act abolished mental hospitals as specially designated hospitals. All patients had the opportunity of being admitted to any hospital able to offer them treatment. All hospitals could offer treatment to any patient they felt they could help and could refuse to admit patients whom they did not feel able to help. Clearly, many hospitals continued to specialize in certain types of treatment and many psychiatric patients required specialized care, but there was no legal restriction on other hospitals or patients.

Most patients suffering from mental disorders were admitted to hospital in precisely the same manner as if they were suffering from any other kind of illness. Only a few patients required to be admitted or detained against their will. Patients who felt that they were wrongfully detained had, however, recourse to specially constituted Mental Health Review Tribunals or, in Scotland, to the Mental Welfare Commission.

The above Acts remained virtually unamended until 1983 (1984 in Scotland). The new Mental Health Acts seek to give the patient greater protection whenever compulsion is involved. Protection of patients has been a matter of deep concern to MIND (National Association for Mental Health)—a voluntary organization which can be justly proud of the fact that many of the new Acts' provisions are based on its proposals. A brief description of the sections of the Acts of particular relevance to psychiatric nurses is given later in the book (see Appendix B).

Investigations into the causes and treatment of psychiatric disorders developed along divergent lines. For example, the chance discovery of malarial therapy for the treatment of so-called general paralysis of the insane (a late manifestation of syphilis) led to a search for organic causes and physical treatment. The first physical treatment—and one still in use today—of value in depressive illness, electroconvulsive therapy (ECT) (see Chapter 13) was introduced in the late 1930s. The breakthrough in psychopharmacology came in 1952 with the first of the antipsychotic agents, chlorpromazine (see Appendix C). Current research in the field of molecular biology is yielding important, if as yet inconclusive, results. Diagnostic imaging is also providing clues to the brain's mental activity, or its non-activity, for example, in the condition loosely known as Alzheimer's disease (also more correctly referred to as senile dementia of the Alzheimer type (SDAT): see Chapter 10), and in dementia associated with AIDS. Research into finding improved drug treatments for psychiatric disorders continues to be carried out.

The importance of this recent biological and genetic research is widely acknowledged by mental health nurses. It requires, however, to be viewed from a wider perspective: Peplau (1990)—the person credited with releasing psychiatric nurses from the shackles of their former custodial role as attendants and guiding them towards embracing their modern function as reflective and knowledgeable practitioners (Carey *et al.*, 1989)—states that by itself this research 'leaves too much out of the equation'. She goes on to warn nurses of the risk they face of losing sight of the unique part they play in meeting clients' psychosocial needs.

The necessity for the nurse to focus care on the person as a whole being with a variety of needs and aspirations, and not solely on a diagnostic 'label', is a feature of the following pages and is reiterated in the philosophy underpinning the human needs model of nursing (see p. 72 below) favoured by the authors.

Investigation of psychological and social causes of mental disorder and treatment by psychotherapy made rapid strides. It was the findings of Freud, the famous psychoanalyst, and his followers which led to increased understanding of personality development and the factors thought to cause faulty adjustment in adulthood. In the 1960s and 1970s the therapeutic community approach to care, as promoted by Dr Maxwell Jones at Dingleton Hospital in Scotland, the concept of social psychiatry, as developed by Dr David Clark at Fulbourn Hospital, Cambridge, and the importance of including meaningful occupation and work in the treatment of people with long-term, severe mental disorder, or industrial therapy, as modelled by Dr Douglas Bennett at the Maudsley Hospital and Dr James Affleck in Scotland, were all crucial components in enabling people with mental disorders to take back more control of their own lives.

The general interest in the prevention of illness which has yielded such marked results in other fields of medicine has spread to psychiatry. There is a widening interest in the social and educational responsibility for developing healthy mental attitudes. Working with families where there is a member with a mental disorder, helping the whole family to understand the issues around the condition, and going into schools to discuss topics that relate to the cause and effect of mental illness are just two ways in which changing attitudes within society indicate its recognition of the need to take its responsibilities towards mental disorder more seriously. Community psychiatric nurses have made a vital contribution in these areas over recent years and are actively involved in many research programmes, seeking for more knowledge on which to base better treatment and management of mental disorder. Mental health promotion has now become an integral part of psychiatric care, in whatever setting. In *The Health of the Nation* (Department of Health, 1992), the Government's White Paper setting out its health strategy for England, it states as one of its main aims that the promotion of healthy living and the prevention of ill-health must be the focus of care for the future.

CURRENT ISSUES IN MENTAL HEALTH

Care in the Community

Since it became government policy, reflecting the change in society's attitude towards mental illness, to encourage the care of people with mental health problems to take place, not in institutions but in the community, many of the old style 'Victorian asylums' have been closed. The patients who had lived there for many years have been discharged into the community, some living in hostels, some living in their own flats or bedsits, some becoming homeless. For many this has been a devastating experience, and although mental health services have believed that they have prepared patients for this fundamental change in their lives, society has not been adequately prepared to receive people back into their communities or to assist in the integration process. As a consequence, many people have found themselves alone in an unwelcoming environment, with few places to go and little to do, on minimum allowances and benefits because they do not know to what they are entitled or how to claim.

Society, in its turn, has become concerned at the apparent speed of hospital closure and lack of appropriate alternative provision for people with long-term, severe mental disorder. Following campaigns in the media and by voluntary organizations such as MIND, National Schizophrenia Fellowship (NSF), SANE (Schizophrenia—A National Emergency) and SHELTER, the Government has produced guidelines on the care of people being discharged into the community, the Care Programme Approach, and has introduced new legislation in the Community Care Act 1990 (Department of Health, 1990). These will be discussed more fully in Chapters 3 and 14. The care of the homeless mentally ill will be considered in Chapter 14 where it belongs as a challenge to the future of psychiatric nursing.

The Incidence and Treatment of Mental Illness among Ethnic Minorities

During the 1980s sociologists and clinicians treating people with mental illness, particularly in inner city areas where there is a preponderance of multi-ethnic communities, began to realize that a disproportionate number of people from an Afro-Caribbean background were being admitted to psychiatric hospitals under a section of the Mental Health Acts and that a large number of these people were being diagnosed as having a schizophrenic illness. The concerns raised by these observations led to research studies to verify and test out theories as to why this was happening. It became clear that the language and behaviour used to describe feelings and thoughts was that which was familiar to black, Afro-Caribbean people, expressing the cultural heritage from which they were descended, but which was unfamiliar to the white, professional clinicians who were responsible for diagnosing and treating them. As these clinicians did not understand what was being expressed to them, and they found some of the ideas and symbolism disturbing, it seemed obvious to them that their patients must be suffering from a distortion of reality and so they must be schizophrenic. The research studies found that these patients were much more likely to be prescribed the physical treatments of drugs and ECT rather than be offered counselling or psychotherapy.

The lessons learned from these studies are that there must be much more effort made to understand the cultural and religious belief systems from which people come, the language and symbolism by which thoughts and feelings are expressed, and for all those who work in the field of mental health to be aware of their own attitudes to race (Ferguson, 1992).

One way of beginning to challenge centuries-old attitudes towards other races and peoples and to begin to understand what is important and meaningful to different peoples is through including race-awareness in training and educational programmes (Fernando, 1991). White workers in the mental health field may well approach the assessment and need for care and treatment, carrying certain assumptions that they take for granted, which may include their own stereotyping of people (Perry, 1992). Research has shown a link between social class, unemployment, poor housing and a greater tendency toward mental illness. Added to these factors are colour and ethnic background and an inability to explain current distress in the way white clinicians can understand. Communications break down on two vital levels: the patient cannot describe the thoughts and feelings being experienced in a way that the doctor, nurse or social worker can understand, and the clinician or social worker cannot put themselves into the position of the patient or client so that they can understand what the other person is experiencing. Thus misunderstandings occur, messages are misinterpreted and people are misdiagnosed.

These problems have been of major concern among the ethnic minorities in Britain, the Asian communities, Afro-Caribbean communities, Chinese and Vietnamese, to name only a few. As the frontiers of the European Union countries are now open there will inevitably be more movement between countries. People will bring their own experiences and expectations from their country of origin. The nuances in language and meaning may be open to misinterpretation. It is essential that all those working in mental health are fully aware of the dangers of too readily interpreting other people's distress in terms that only hold meaning for their own experience and background.

SUMMARY

This chapter has provided a brief review of the history of the care and treatment of people with psychiatric illnesses in the light of contemporary knowledge and attitudes. It has traced that history from the days in which people were shut away in asylums and regarded as creatures to be feared and restrained, through the enlightened approach of doctors in France and England who encouraged and developed a more humane attitude, to the increased interest in searching for causes and explanations for mental illness through research. This has resulted in new approaches and new drug treatments enabling people with mental disorders no longer to face years in hospital but to return to more fulfilling and meaningful lives in the community. This in itself has posed new questions and concerns for society which has yet to reach a satisfactory balance in both its attitude to the care of people with mental health problems and the way in which it provides care for people with mental health problems.

FURTHER READING

Brooking J, Ritter S & Thomas B (eds) (1992) *A Textbook of Psychiatric and Mental Health Nursing*. Edinburgh: Churchill Livingstone.

Community Relations Commission (1976) *Aspects of Mental Health in a Multi-Cultural Society*. London: Community Relations Commission.

Khan VS (1979) *Minority Families in Britain: Support and Stress*. London: Macmillan Press.

Littlewood R & Lipsedge M (1982) *Aliens and Alienists: Ethnic Minorities and Psychiatry*, 2nd edn. London: Unwin Hyman.

Mercer K (1896) Racism and trans-cultural psychiatry. In: Miller P & Rose N *The Power of Psychiatry*. London: Polity Press.

Sashidharan S (1989) *Schizophrenia or Just Black?* Community Care 5/10/1989.

REFERENCES

Carey E, Noll J, Ramussen I *et al.* (1989) Hildegard Peplau: Psychodynamic nursing. In: Marriner-Tomy A (ed.) *Nurse Theorists and Their Work*, 2nd edn. St Louis: Mosby.

Department of Health (1990) *NHS Reforms and Community Care Act 1990*. London: HMSO.

Department of Health (1992) *The Health of the Nation*. HMSO: London.

Ferguson G (1992) Race and mental health. *Community Psychiatric Nursing Journal*, **12**(6): 11–17.

Fernando S (1991) *Mental Health, Race and Culture*. London: Macmillan.

Peplau H (1990) Interpersonal relations: principles and general applications. In: Reynolds W & Cormack D (eds) *Psychiatric and Mental Health Nursing: Theory and Practice.* London: Chapman and Hall.

Perry F (1992) Black and white issues. *Nursing Times* **88**(10): 62–64.

SECTION II: ORGANIZATION OF CARE

Chapter 3
Community Practice

INTRODUCTION

Chapter 2 explored developments in care and treatment and their effects on patients. With the increasing enlightenment of society, and its change in attitude towards people suffering from mental illnesses or emotional disorders, came new discoveries in drugs. These helped to reduce and control many of the symptoms of illness and disorder with which families and society could not cope. These two factors helped to make it possible for hospital staff to take the risk of allowing patients to spend more and more time outside hospital, back in the communities in which they lived with their families before being admitted to hospital. This chapter examines the impact of this on the organization of care.

THE DEVELOPMENT OF COMMUNITY PSYCHIATRIC NURSING

In 1954 the first community psychiatric nurses (CPNs) were appointed at Warlingham Park, Surrey, with a specific brief to visit patients who had been discharged from hospital. Their role was to see how patients were coping with everyday life and to check that any medication which had been prescribed was being taken and was not producing any unwanted side-effects. They were also able to give support and encouragement to families and relatives who may have been anxious about how to manage the patients' behaviour.

From this simple, but highly significant, beginning has developed the modern practice of community psychiatric nursing. Psychiatric nurses have taken the skills learned in their traditional, hospital-based training and adapted them to the needs of their patients or clients who now live in the community. They have discovered that, as nurses visiting people in their homes, meeting other members of the family, seeing the circumstances in which their patients live, they have had to develop other skills and to become much more resourceful and imaginative in meeting the needs of their clients.

Other factors also influenced the development of CPN services from those early beginnings.

- The implementation of the recommendations of the Seebohm Report (1968) which changed the role of the specialist psychiatric social worker into that of a generic social worker, leaving a gap in the provision of rehabilitation and social care for those who were being resettled into the community.
- The publication of the Government White Paper, *Better Services for the Mentally Ill* (Department of Health and Social Security, 1975) which recognized the need to develop more flexible services that were more accessible to local communities and considered the needs of those with both long-term and short-term illnesses. It encouraged specialist mental health teams to

work closely with primary health care teams, with CPNs providing a significant contribution to the care of people with mental health problems in the community.

• The decision to run down the large psychiatric institutions built in the Victorian era, with plans to close many of them, and to resettle most or all of the long-term patients in the community.

Nowadays, people usually spend a tiny proportion of their lives in hospital. Much the greater part is spent *outside* hospital, in the community. The Government is encouraging health authorities and social services to concentrate resources where people actually live, and to make it possible for them to receive the treatment and care that they need with as little disruption to themselves and their families as possible. This is not to say that there may not be occasions when a period in hospital is desirable, or even essential, for the safety and well-being of the individual or for society, as, for example, when someone feels like killing himself, or when thoughts are so disordered that a person feels compelled to harm someone else. However, admission to hospital is now usually seen as one part of a *continuum* of care which may begin before admission and continue after discharge.

Growth of Community Psychiatric Nursing Services

During the second half of the 1970s CPN services grew rapidly, both in terms of new services in health districts and in terms of an increase in numbers within services. This led to the development of specialist services for distinct client groups, such as the elderly, children and adolescents, those with alcohol or drug problems, and for the rehabilitation and resettlement of those who had been in hospital for many years, and also, in some areas, crisis intervention teams.

The Community Psychiatric Nurses' Association has carried out a survey every five years since 1980 which has looked at a number of issues such as the organization of CPN services, the degree of specialization, the pattern of care, the proportion of 'trained' to untrained CPNs (meaning the percentage of the total CPN workforce that has completed a post-registration course in community psychiatric nursing) (Community (Psychiatric Nurses' Association, 1980, 1985; White, 1991). The results of these three surveys show an increase in the total number of CPNs from 1667 (1980), to 2758 (1985), to 4351 (1990), reflecting the very rapid growth and development of community psychiatric nursing since its beginnings in 1954.

Recognition of the Need to Develop a Wider Skills Base

All the early CPN services began from within psychiatric hospitals, with the CPN being a member of a team of professionals providing care to a geographically designated area. Referrals were usually received from the medical members of that team. Gradually, one or two services began to experiment with placing CPNs in locally based health centres, working alongside the members of the primary care team, taking their referrals from any member of that team. This practice soon led CPNs to recognize that they needed to learn new skills to help the clients who were being referred to them. Some of these people presented with histories of long-term disabilities that had affected the quality of their lives over long periods of time.

- Their relationships with different members of their families had contributed to their present difficulties, usually due to an inability to speak openly and honestly together; family members often colluded in keeping individuals locked in their disability, forcing them to adopt a 'sick role' rather than face the family problem. This led to a need to develop skills in working with families.

- Many people presented with fears and anxiety, leading to panic attacks, which severely affected their ability to lead full, active, satisfying lives. CPNs recognized the need to work in a more behavioural style, using skills and techniques that they learned from their behaviour nurse therapist colleagues.

- In all their contacts they recognized the importance of developing counselling skills, to a greater level of sophistication and expertise than they had learned in their original training, whether they were caring for the depressed person, someone who had been bereaved, a parent who was coming to terms with a child being diagnosed as having schizophrenia, or any one of a multiplicity of reasons.

- More and more frequently, CPNs were discovering that a significant number of the people being referred to them revealed a history of sexual abuse in childhood which had affected the way they coped in later life. CPNs recognized how ill-equipped they were to help these people in their distress and began to seek training and supervision to enable them to work more effectively and sensitively with their clients. (See Chapter 13 for a fuller discussion of some of the skills practised by nurses.)

Current Issues

More recently, the Government has reacted to the public outcry of seeing more people wandering aimlessly around towns and cities, particularly seaside resorts, with nowhere to go and nothing to do, sometimes ending up sleeping rough and becoming homeless. These people were among those who had been relocated or rehoused as hospitals were preparing to close, but with no proper provision for their aftercare or follow-up. Often they stopped taking their prescribed medication and relapsed, requiring readmission to hospital. This could become problematical as fewer and fewer hospital places are available. Smaller acute services were incorporated into district general hospitals (DGHs) which were less able to cater for the needs of this group of people. This led to a number of policy statements from the Department of Health such as:

- *Discharge of Patients from Hospital* (Department of Health, 1989a)
- *The Care Programme Approach for People with a Mental Illness Referred to the Specialist Psychiatric Services* (Department of Health, 1990)
- Community Care Act 1990
- *Caring for People—Community Care in the Next Decade and Beyond* (Department of Health, 1989b)

These policy statements drew attention to the aftercare needs of patients discharged into the community. This will be discussed in more detail later in the chapter.

THE ROLE OF THE COMMUNITY PSYCHIATRIC NURSE

When community psychiatric nursing became an established and recognized discipline, requiring a distinct training course accredited by the Joint Board of Clinical Nursing Studies in 1975, CPNs began to try to define their role and function. This has been a contentious issue among CPNs for many years. Carr, Butterworth and Hodges (1980) in the first attempt to make a clear statement of what CPNs do suggested six main areas:

1 the CPN as a *clinician*
2 the CPN as an *assessor*
3 the CPN as a *therapist*
4 the CPN as an *educator*
5 the CPN as a *resource*
6 the CPN as a *consultant*

These six categories include aspects of what CPNs do and continue to provide a framework for CPNs, but over the last 10 years or so the emphasis has changed, as the needs and demands of society and policy have changed. Simmons and Brooker (1986) discussed the two main directions in which CPN services could develop in the later stages of the 1980s:

- into 'primary health care, health education and the prevention of mental ill-health';
- into 'community care for the residents of psychiatric hospitals, many of whom have been in hospital for a large part of their adult lives'.

They quote the Social Services Select Committee (1985): 'The CPN is probably the most important single professional in the process of moving care of mental illness into the community.'

CPNs have an important contribution in both these areas, taking their knowledge and expertise into primary care where the great majority of people with psychological and emotional problems are seen, but at the same time providing the core of the care and support to people with long-term mental health problems, alongside family members and those who provide sheltered accommodation outside hospitals.

CPNs and the Nursing Process

CPNs along with most other nurses, use the principles of the nursing process to organize the care that they give:

- Assessment
- Planning
- Implementation
- Evaluation (see Chapter 4)

Carrying out a thorough mental health assessment of a client's needs is one of the most important roles of a CPN. It includes:

- defining and agreeing what the problems are;
- considering the present family structure and circumstances;
- considering the client's work situation;
- exploring the client's network of relationships and support available;
- finding out what contact the client already has with doctors and what medication, if any, has been prescribed;
- taking as full a history as possible to assess the mental state of the client.

Most CPN services have devised a set of guidelines which provide a framework on which to make the assessment. This is an essential activity before any plan of action can be agreed. It has been shown that for a treatment programme to be successful the agreement and cooperation of the client, and, where appropriate, significant relatives and friends, is an important pre-requisite.

What the CPN actually plans and how that plan is implemented will clearly depend on what problem areas have been identified. The interventions agreed together may be of a short-term nature, such as:

- engaging in an anxiety management treatment pro-gramme which runs for six to eight weeks;
- short-term counselling for a specific number of sessions;
- help and support through a particular crisis.

They may be of a more practical nature such as:

- providing advice and help in finding more suitable accommodation;
- making arrangements for collecting benefits at the local post office;
- attending an outpatient appointment.

In the case of those people who have been resettled into the community after years in hospitals, the CPN's role may be in:

- supporting them, over many years, in adjusting to the demands of life outside hospital;
- encouraging them to develop greater independence and confidence in themselves;
- helping them to integrate into the community into which they have moved, maintaining whatever level of ability they have.

CPNs may work with clients on an individual basis, or may work with them in conjunction with others, with couples, with families or in larger groups of eight or ten people with similar difficulties, such as in social skills groups, relaxation and anxiety management groups, or in supportive 'talking' groups, where people meet to talk through their difficult feelings and at the same time offer support to one another.

CPNs often work alongside other professionals or with voluntary organizations in providing informal 'drop-in' facilities where people can call in, knowing that there will be a warm welcome, a cup of tea, and an opportunity to raise an issue of concern, or sort out a practical problem that is causing distress. CPNs come to know their 'patch' very well, building up their own network of contacts so that they can put their clients in touch with people or organizations which best fit their individual needs. Some areas have developed 'befriending schemes' which enable those who may have lost confidence through their illness to make ordinary, normal contact with everyday things once more, with the help of an accepting, non-professional friend, who may also help them to resume old interests or explore new ones. The CPN's role in these areas is to know about the various facilities available and to be able to put clients in touch with them.

CPNs and Health Education and Health Promotion

Whatever the type of intervention, nurses, whether they work in hospital settings, day care settings or community settings, will find themselves involved in health education in some form or another. It may be through helping people to understand the importance of eating a healthy diet at regular intervals and the link between nutrition, medication and a healthy mind. It may be teaching people relaxation exercises and mechanisms to cope with anxiety. It may be helping relatives to learn to manage the odd behaviour or accept the mannerisms of the client, or how to express their own feelings in support groups. It may be in giving formal teaching sessions to local groups about what is and what is not mental illness. The list and the opportunities are endless. All nurses, including CPNs, now see health education as an important, integral part of their role and welcome any opportunity to enable people to understand health and illness, and to help them to lead healthier lives.

CPNs learned very early the importance of liaison in their work. In order not to engage in wasteful duplication of time and effort they recognized that they must keep their professional colleagues informed as to what they were doing and to seek information from them whenever relevant. Now that the Care Programme Approach and the Community Care Act require a named care coordinator or care manager, CPNs who have often been performing this role in an unofficial capacity are able to fulfil the duties of care coordination relatively easily.

Education

The role of the CPN as an educator has been mentioned in the context of patient and client care. It is important to remember that they have a central role in the training of student nurses. At present there are two training courses running.

1 The last groups of students to train under the 1982 syllabus will complete their courses within the next year.
2 Project 2000 has been running since 1989 in England and was introduced in Scotland in the autumn of 1992.

It is hoped that Project 2000 will provide the opportunity for mental health nurse training to become more community based, with students spending a significant proportion of their time in the community, learning about the sociological concepts of 'community', the demographic needs of a community with its 'health profile', how service planners decide which services are to be developed, as well as learning how to deliver care to people to fulfil their health care needs.

CPNs are involved in the supervision of students as they learn and develop their skills in a much more active way than perhaps previously. Students come to the community having had less practical experience on hospital wards, so it is hoped that they will begin to think in terms of the whole person, see clients in the context of their own homes, relating to families and friends, struggling with their own particular social constraints and circumstances. Students should be able to experience at first hand all the different areas that CPNs take into account when assessing a person's needs, along with assessing that person's mental state. Students should actually see the degree of strain that relatives experience when there is a mentally ill person in the family. They will observe the cooperation and liaison that occurs between members of the primary care team and the Community Mental Health Team. They may take part in initiating treatment programmes, in researching what other facilities are available in an area. If necessary, they may follow a client's progress from the community into hospital and back home again.

Although CPNs have increased opportunities to influence the training of student nurses, their own training needs are as important. The three quinquennial surveys carried out by the Community Psychiatric Nurses' Association (1980, 1985; White, 1991) show that only a proportion of CPNs practising at any one time have received any specific training in caring for people with mental health problems in the community. The community education and practice proposals from the UKCC (1991) suggested that all nurses working in the community should receive training before being allowed to practise in the community. There should be a common core programme for all nurses, with modules for the specific areas of health visiting, community nursing, school nursing, community psychiatric nursing, community mental handicap nursing. Some Colleges of Further Education have held joint modules with social work students, so encouraging a greater understanding of the different roles, and helping to lessen the tension between the different disciplines.

However, the UKCC, in the final draft of its report *The Future of Professional Practice and Education* (1993) has not been so specific. Community psychiatric nursing is accepted as an area of specialist practice, along with all the other current branches of community nursing which together comprise 'community health care nursing'. To qualify in one of these specialist areas of practice nurses will be required to complete an education course of at least six months which will be taught in modules and will consist of equal components of theory and practice. The course can be completed either in a six month block or spread over a maximum period of five years. These arrangements have yet to be finally approved. As students graduate from the Project 2000 courses, CPN training courses will need to change, becoming more skills-based, to equip nurses working in the community to respond effectively to the needs of clients who are referred to their care.

Supervision

As CPNs have felt the need to learn new skills in order to respond to the needs of their clients so they have recognized the importance of receiving supervision for their work with clients. The term 'supervision' as used here means having the opportunity to meet regularly with someone to examine what is happening in the relationship between the CPN and the client and so increase self-awareness and confidence, to assist in developing skills and recognizing good practice. This 'clinical supervision' may be achieved on a variety of levels.

- Through peer supervision when a group of CPNs meets together to discuss the progress of an individual's care, making suggestions, providing support, helping to sort out particularly tricky problems.
- Through supervision on an individual basis from a colleague who is a specialist in a particular skill or technique, such as a nurse behaviour therapist or someone who practises as a family therapist.
- CPNs who work in multidisciplinary teams may have team supervision when members of the team meet to examine the dynamics of working together and how this may be affecting the success or failure of a treatment programme of an individual client.

CPN managers have a role to play in helping CPNs to manage and organize their time and their caseload so that they are able to make the most efficient and effective use of their working day, in other words 'management supervision'. In all these areas the main aim of supervision is to enable the CPN to be a safe, competent practitioner.

MULTIDISCIPLINARY TEAM APPROACH TO CARE

Teams

Regardless of the setting in which the individual person is treated, 'teamwork' is a concept that the learner will often hear discussed and will see in action. The idea of the multidisciplinary team approach to care is that different groups of people with professional training and expertise work together for the benefit of people with mental health problems. If the care is being delivered in a hospital setting the team may be called the Ward Team or the Sector Team. If the care is being delivered in the community it will be called the Community Mental Health Team. Frequently the members of each team may overlap by working in both settings but the professional disciplines represented will normally consist of one or more of the following:

- consultant psychiatrist
- nurse
- psychologist
- occupational therapist
- arts therapist (music, art, drama)
- social worker
- mental health worker
- secretary

In both settings there will be the 'core' members, as listed above, and there will be other workers whose contribution is vital to the successful delivery of the care needed by each individual. In hospital, other members of the 'extended' team may include the ward domestic staff, the ward clerks, the hospital chaplain, the recreational therapist, the pharmacist, the hospital porters, the telephonists, all of whom may have more or less direct contact with patients (Pollock, 1986). In the community, especially in the case of teams who work with the elderly, the 'extended' team may include a physiotherapist and a chiropodist.

The Role of the Nurse in the Multidisciplinary Team

The nurse has a key role in the multidisciplinary team as the overall coordinator of care. In a psychiatric unit, as in other inpatient facilities, this duty devolves on the nurse because of the 24 hour, round-the-clock contact with the patient. Furthermore, this continuing presence provides the nurse with an ideal opportunity to form a relationship with the patients in her care. It places her in a unique position to assess their changing needs and to report the changes and progress in their emotional, physical, cognitive and social conditions.

In the role as coordinator the nurse frequently has occasion to liaise with other team members. For example, a young girl in her late teens, emerging from a severe depressive episode, may disclose to a nurse one evening that she is worried about losing the secretarial skills she learned at college shortly before coming to hospital. With the patient's consent, the nurse subsequently raises the concern with the multidisciplinary team, who agree that if it is in the patient's best interests, the occupational therapist will make arrangements for the girl to use the word processing equipment in the occupational therapy department.

The Benefits of Teamwork and Working Together

As well as promoting improved intra-team communication by the sharing of knowledge and information which can lead to the provision of practical help for the patient, as illustrated above, teamwork also prevents unnecessary confusion in the patient by ensuring consistency of approach and continuity of care. Efficient and optimum patient care should follow, which is, of course, the ultimate goal of multidisciplinary teamwork. Multidisciplinary team meetings are held regularly, whether on the ward or in the community, when team members have the opportunity to share information, exchange experiences and ideas freely and allow for decisions to be made, based on all available information. Considerable effort on the part of each team member is necessary for the effective functioning of the team. Only by working closely together can members learn more about each other's roles, particular areas of interest and expertise. Recognition of the skills of other members, a willingness to negotiate and the ability to be flexible all make a substantial contribution towards efficiency in working together as a team and to the avoidance of unnecessary duplication of time and energy.

Difficulties within the team can sometimes arise, however, and two of the issues which may militate against harmonious teamwork are now briefly considered.

Leadership of the Team

Who should lead the multidisciplinary team? Traditionally this has been the role of the consultant psychiatrist. Leadership depends to some extent on the setting in which care takes place. The charge nurse of a unit devoted to caring for elderly mentally ill people is eminently suited to lead that team. In a rehabilitation unit where behavioural therapy techniques are used the clinical psychologist may be the leader of choice. In both these settings the psychiatrist has to be prepared to relinquish the traditional leadership role assigned to him in the past by virtue of the legal responsibilities for patients in his care.

The style of leadership can affect the way the team functions. Team members can feel marginalized and frustrated if decisions are imposed on them by an autocratic leader who leaves little or no room for dialogue or dissent. On the other hand a leader who is too democratic and indecisive can lead to too much discussion and not enough action.

The team leader must be someone who commands the respect of the other members of the team and who has the authority to make sure that the decisions reached are implemented. Leading a team includes making time available for team-building, allowing members to speak openly and frankly, giving encouragement and praise when deserved and providing constructive advice and support when people may be feeling concerned about their clinical work. Good, firm, clear leadership will contribute greatly to keeping morale high, to maintaining motivation, towards facilitating open communication channels and, ultimately, to ensuring high quality effective care to clients, their carers and the community at large.

Interdisciplinary Conflicts

Interdisciplinary conflicts are more likely to arise in a team led by an autocratic leader than in one whose leader favours a democratic and egalitarian style, permitting members to express their views freely, in the knowledge that their contributions will be valued. Conflicts frequently occur if insufficient time is taken to ascertain and acknowledge the special skills of each team member and may persist unless participants are able to meet together frequently to air their grievances openly in an informal and supportive atmosphere. As mentioned above, this can be dealt with through taking active measures to build a team identity in which each person recognizes the knowledge and skills that every other member brings to the team. There may be areas where skills overlap: nurses and occupational therapists use the skills developed by psychologists when they engage in behaviour therapy programmes with clients; social workers and nurses may use their knowledge of the benefits system for helping clients to cope with their financial affairs; CPNs may advise general practitioners (GPs) on matters of medication if they have more frequent contact with the primary care team than the psychiatrist is able to have. Skills are not necessarily mutually exclusive, but by recognizing who has the expert knowledge and experience, skills can be shared to the benefit of clients.

Community Mental Health Teams

The Community Mental Health Team is a method of delivering care that is spreading throughout the country. The organization of these teams may vary from district to district, but the principle remains that of a multidisciplinary approach to provide care to people as close to their homes as possible. As has been discussed above, the teams will usually consist of core members and others, depending on the needs of each individual person. Their main tasks are, with the cooperation of their colleagues in the primary health care teams:

- GPs
- district nurses

- health visitors
- school nurses
- community midwives

to identify people showing signs of mental illness, or emotional disorder, or confusion as early as possible so that treatment can begin at an early stage of the illness, and, wherever possible, prevent further or unnecessary deterioration or disturbance.

As with every other condition, people suffering from mental health problems may require intervention only once in their lives; but those who have severe, or major, mental illness will experience periods when they are comparatively well and able to cope with their daily lives, interspersed with periods when their symptoms become much more active. These symptoms interfere with their work, affect their relationships and their ability to care for themselves. With the regular contact from the mental health workers of the Community Mental Health Teams it should be possible to intervene quickly and to encourage people to receive the treatment needed to prevent further deterioration. It may be necessary to encourage them to go into hospital voluntarily, or informally, for a short time only, and to return home as quickly as possible, thus reducing the disruption to the rest of the family as much as possible.

CPNs and the Mental Health Acts

Sadly, there will be times when people refuse to accept that they are becoming ill. They refuse to take any medication or to consider an increase or change in medication, but they cannot be described in the terms of the Mental Health Acts as being a danger to themselves or to others.

In these situations families and staff have little chance of helping these people until they become disturbed enough to require admission under a section of the Mental Health Act (see Appendix B). Social workers are obliged to consider all alternatives to compulsory admission in order to protect individuals' rights not to be detained unless absolutely necessary. It can be a most humiliating experience and give rise to complex feelings of guilt and shame in all concerned, so, great skill and sensitivity needs to be learned when managing admissions under a section of the Mental Health Act.

CPNs do not have an active role in the formalities of 'sectioning' people, but they do have a crucial role in giving advice and support to the patient, their carers, and to their professional colleagues, as it is so often the CPN who knows the patient/client best, through the relationship that has grown over the months and years from regular contact.

Every effort is made by the Community Mental Health Team to avoid admission unless absolutely necessary. Some mental health services have specific crisis intervention teams which work intensively with families throughout the crisis, gradually reducing the amount of involvement as things settle down and are resolved.

COMMUNITY CARE PROGRAMME APPROACH

This requires health and social services to collaborate together in order to ensure that care is provided to the most vulnerable group of people who are at risk of losing contact, relapsing and requiring readmission to hospital.

- Policies and procedures are to be agreed by which it is known who requires the Care Programme Approach (CPA).
- At a pre-discharge meeting a care coordinator is agreed who will be responsible for seeing that the care programme, or care package agreed by the multidisciplinary team, is actually carried out.
- The care coordinator will be responsible for calling a review meeting at regular intervals to reassess each person's needs.
- The care coordinator is the named person with whom other workers, the family and carers, or any people involved with that person, can be in touch. The care coordinator does not necessarily carry out all the care for that individual, but ensures that everyone is responsible for their particular part of the care package agreed for any particular individual.
- A register is to be kept of all people included on the Care Programme Approach so that they can be easily monitored and services can carry out their own auditing to see how successfully the system is responding to the needs of this vulnerable group in any locality.
- Although the Government has nominated the local authority as the budget-holder for providing appropriate resources for the care of people with serious mental health problems living in the community, it is very clear that there is much inter-linkage between health and social needs for people with mental health problems, so the assessment processes for deciding need have to be done on a joint basis, respecting each other's professional skills and experience, and involving both the individual person and their carers wherever possible.
- The guidelines for this process include encouraging the use of facilities developed in the voluntary and

independent sectors, whether in housing, day care provision, social clubs, and so on.
- Health services are to concentrate on providing assessment, diagnosis and treatment with an emphasis on the prevention of illness and the promotion of health through supporting primary care.

COMMUNITY CARE ACT 1990

The Attitude of Society

Social attitudes have been changing for many years, with increasing concern at the custodial care meted out to people with mental health problems in the past. However, society in general is still not comfortable with accepting people back into the community and learning how to contribute to their integration, or reintegration, after an episode in hospital. The media and voluntary organizations have championed the cause of those who have been discharged from hospital without adequate provision being made for their needs or supervision of their care. The rush to close outdated and outmoded hospitals which were built as asylums in the middle of the nineteenth century outran the ability or will to provide proper alternative resources and facilities. People who had known only the protected environment of the hospital and its grounds were ill-prepared to cope with life in society, and society was not prepared to cope with those who had so conveniently been cared for in institutions. It is only in the last fifty years or so, since the end of the Second World War, that hospitals began to open their doors. With advances in medication, it became possible to control symptoms, so that people suffering from delusions and hallucinations could lead more normal lives without so much fear of violent and apparently uncontrolled behaviour.

The NHS and Community Care Act 1990 tries to set statutory standards to address many of the problems that have emerged over the last few years. The idea of hospital care, or asylum in its true sense, is being recognized as a part of a continuum of care, when all aspects of a person's needs are considered. A named care coordinator becomes responsible for ensuring that all agencies involved in any one person's care know their own and everyone else's part in delivering that care, so that fewer people are left to become lost, homeless, drifting aimlessly with little to do and nowhere to go.

Attitude of Professionals

All people working in the mental health field are being required to rethink some of their assumptions. One of the most fundamental changes is that of involving clients and their carers in deciding what treatment and care is necessary and desirable. For so long professionals believed that they knew best what was right for individuals, without listening to relatives or even to the patient. Professionals are now recognizing that carers who have lived with members of their family as they became ill, who have seen behaviours change and who have been part of events that may well have contributed to breakdown, have an essential role in enabling recovery and reintegration into life and must be taken on as partners in the treatment and caring role.

The Patient's Charter, published by the Department of Health (1991), states that people have a right to be given all information about treatment and possible alternatives to treatment before any decision is made. Proper arrangements have to be made before discharge from hospital if it is decided that care will be needed outside hospital. All relevant people must be involved in planning care and this includes the patient and their carers.

Although mental health services have for many years been working to enable people with long-term mental health problems to live in the community there has been much criticism that these people have been left to fend for themselves without adequate help. Sufficient resources have not been devolved or developed into the community to cater for the needs of this particularly vulnerable group of people who may have been living in hospitals for many years, or who may have lost the skills that normally healthy people take for granted in coping with the everyday tasks of life. The new community care legislation is the Government's attempt to address these issues.

The aims of the reforms are to enable vulnerable people to live as independently as possible in their own homes or in a homely setting in the community.

The White Paper, *Caring for People* (Department of Health, 1989b), sets out how this is to be achieved.

- The development of the right services to help people live in their own homes wherever this is possible and sensible.
- Making sure that those who provide services give high priority to giving carers practical support.
- Proper assessment of need and good case management are the cornerstones of high quality care.
- The development of a flourishing independent sector alongside good quality public provision.
- Health and social services are clear about their

responsibilities and promote better coordination in providing services.
- Better value for money in providing care.

The Act makes social services the lead authority and gives them the funding to provide for the care of the most vulnerable groups of people living in the community. There has been a requirement on local social service departments since 1992 to produce a community care plan based on the assessment of the needs of the local population. This plan has to be reviewed each year and any changes published. One of the most significant changes is that from April 1993 any person who has complex social or residential needs is assessed by social services.

The following areas must always be considered when caring for people with long-term mental health problems in the community.

- Housing arrangements which may be in a supported hostel, group home, bedsit, independent flat or at home with parents and family.
- Daytime activities which could involve full-time work, sheltered work, attendance at day hospital or day centre, or a combination which is tailor-made to fit each person's individual needs.
- Recreational and leisure activities which could include calling in at drop-in centres, social clubs, sporting activities, community education classes, all the things that most people like to do outside their working day.
- Most importantly, consideration and attention must be given to the support networks for each person, so that they and their carers know to whom they may turn when things begin to look worrying.

Much more emphasis is now being given to making sure both patients and their carers have access to the information they need about the illness, about the treatment and medication they are expected to take, about the range and accessibility of services and facilities available, and whom to contact in times of trouble.

Much of the rest of this book looks at how current knowledge and expertise is being applied to enable people to live out of hospitals and institutions and to prevent them from becoming institutionalized and cut off from the practicalities of living in the real world. It is to be hoped that experience gained over the last few years will help those planning the services of the future so that the same mistakes are not repeated to the detriment of those suffering from severe, long-term mental illness.

SUMMARY

This chapter has been concerned with the development of community psychiatric nursing, from its earliest days, when nurses went out from hospital to visit newly discharged patients in their own homes, to the present, when CPNs have increased and developed their skills to respond to the varied needs of the people referred to them. Nurses are seen to be members of multidisciplinary teams whether in hospital or community settings. The ways in which the changing attitudes of society have influenced the delivery of care have been explored, resulting in the Community Care Act and the Care Programme Approach which attempt to ensure that the needs of people with long-term mental illness are properly planned and provided for.

FURTHER READING

Simmons S & Brooker C (1986) *Community Psychiatric Nursing—A Social Perspective*. London: Heinemann Nursing.

REFERENCES

Carr P, Butterworth CA & Hodges BE (1980) *Community Psychiatric Nursing*. Edinburgh: Churchill-Livingstone.

Community Psychiatric Nurses' Association (1980) *National Survey of Community Psychiatric Nursing Services*. Leeds: CPNA Publications.

Community Psychiatric Nurses' Association (1985) *The 1985 CPNA National Survey Update*. Leeds: CPNA Publications.

Department of Health (1989a) *Discharge of Patients from Hospital*. London: HMSO.

Department of Health (1989b) *Caring for People—Community Care in the Next Decade and Beyond*. London: HMSO.

Department of Health (1990) *The Care Programme Approach for People with a Mental Illness Referred to the Specialist Psychiatric Services*, HC[90]23/LASSL[90]11. London: HMSO.

Department of Health (1991) *The Patient's Charter*. London: HMSO.

Department of Health (1992) *The Health of the Nation*. London: HMSO.

Department of Health and Social Security (1975) *Better Services for the Mentally Ill*. London: HMSO.

Pollock, L (1986) The Multidisciplinary Team. In: Hume C & Pullen I (eds) *Rehabilitation in Psychiatry*. Edinburgh: Churchill Livingstone.

Simmons S & Brooker C (1986) *Community Psychiatric Nursing—A Social Perspective*. London: Heinemann Nursing.

UKCC (1991) *The Report on Proposals for the Future of Community Education and Practice*. London: UKCC.

UKCC (1993) *The Future of Professional Practice and Education*. London: UKCC.

White E (1991) *Community Psychiatric Nursing: The 1990 National Survey*. Nuneaton: Community Psychiatric Nurses' Association Publications.

Chapter 4
Organization of Nursing Care

INTRODUCTION

Almost three decades have passed since it was suggested that for further improvements to take place in the quality of patient care, nursing practice required more than simply a reliance on intuition and experience.

The first calls for a more rational and systematic assessment of the needs of individual patients came from nurses working in the US. A few years later pleas were answered with the *nursing process*, also known as *a systematic approach to care*—a new way of looking at the practice of nursing with particular emphasis on the patient as a unique individual.

Primary nursing and *models of nursing* have since followed (discussed later in this chapter); all three innovations can be seen as examples of important contributions to the development of a distinctive nursing practice underpinned by a firm theoretical base and the demise of nursing's image as the handmaiden of the medical profession.

THE NURSING PROCESS: A SYSTEMATIC APPROACH TO CARE

Stages of the Nursing Process

The nursing process may be divided into stages, exemplifying the systematic step-by-step approach used when caring for each individual patient. The four stages are as follows.

1 Assessment of the patient
2 Planning care
3 Implementation or delivery of the planned care
4 Evaluation of the care given

1 Assessment of the Patient

Assessment is crucial to the concept of the nursing process. It is a systematic method of collecting information about an individual, interpreting and evaluating this information. Minshull *et al.* (1986) add that unless nurses have a 'model of nursing from which to develop a framework for assessment' the information sought and collected may be irrelevant and of little value: not only is this time-wasting, it is an intrusion into a person's privacy. Accurate assessment ensures that each person's unique set of psychological, physical, social and spiritual needs for nursing can be identified and that the care given is effective.

At this point the need to set priorities should be mentioned. For example, during the assessment of a severely depressed person the physical need for a safe environment and possibly for adequate nutrition, if unmet, could be life threatening and so take precedence over other needs. With each reassessment of the person's needs, priorities can be changed as appropriate.

In a community setting the sources of information, as well as the individual, could include:

• the general practitioner
• the referring agent
• relatives

- accompanying friends
- other members of the community team

During the assessment process the CPN's observations of the person's responses and overall mental state will play an important part. The CPN will also be taking into account the circumstances that make up an individual's lifestyle: home, work, relationships, leisure activities.

In order for a full assessment of the person's needs to take place when admitted to hospital, members of the multidisciplinary care team are also involved. However, irrespective of the care setting the amount and nature of the information a person reveals can depend on the interviewer's reactions. If a person notices that, for example, the nurse feels upset, disgusted, disapproving, there will be an immediate censorship on what is being revealed. Thus the extent to which a person is able to open up and permit the nurse to assess his difficulties depends on whether or not he perceives the nurse to be genuinely interested, concerned and non-judgemental.

The nature of the information obtained for assessment purposes will also depend on the patient's state of mind. If the person, on admission to hospital, is very depressed and withdrawn, or excitable and overactive, an initial assessment may be made mainly from the nurses' observations and from other supplementary sources such as relatives and friends. But, whenever practicable, the admitting nurse—the patient's primary nurse or key worker (see p. 62)—will invite the new patient to be interviewed, to get a fuller picture of him or her as a unique individual. Further interviews may be needed to complete the assessment, preferably within the next few days.

The use of a structured assessment form for the comprehensive and systematic gathering of information about patients admitted to acute psychiatric wards has been researched by Tissier (1986) and Mulhearn (1989). They found this tool particularly useful in generating psychosocial problems experienced by patients. Learners especially liked this approach to assessment; they felt it helped towards forming a relationship with a new patient. The opportunity afforded by this method for extensive interaction with a nurse seemed more than adequately to compensate the patient for any anxieties aroused by the questions themselves.

Brooker and Baguley (1990) recommend a structured form known as the Schizophrenia: Nursing Assessment Protocol (SNAP) for use by CPNs and other mental health workers when making a comprehensive psychosocial assessment, not only of the person suffering from schizophrenia but also of the carers involved. Data collected are used to plan care focused on the reduction of stress in both groups of individuals.

The final stages of the initial assessment of the patient may not be concluded until, as has been said, further interviews have taken place, nor until the nurse has had occasion to be with the patient in a variety of situations. It may not be possible to know, for example, that a patient feels very angry about the way he has been treated by his son until the topic of family dynamics has cropped up in, say, a group therapy session or in a one-to-one conversation with a nurse. Initial assessments, however, quickly become dated. Reassessment is required in the light of the person's ever-changing needs.

Information about an individual can also be obtained from *observation* and the following aspects will be discussed.

- Observational skills
- Cultural differences in behaviour
- Abnormal behaviour in psychiatric disorders

- Participant observation and observer effect
- Objectivity
- Bias and selectively
- Recording and reporting observations

Observational skills. An integral part of the nursing assessment of the person in need of care is the ability of the
nurse to make full use of observational skills (Barker,
1986; Ironbar & Hooper, 1989). As soon as the nurse
meets the newcomer she attends closely to how he
presents himself, to what he says and does. For example,
the nurse first of all may note from the person's general
appearance that he has been neglecting personal care; his
face is unshaven, his clothes are in need of ironing. She
may then draw the inference that this person has lost all
interest in himself and in how he appears to others and
conclude that perhaps he is depressed. Although this is
not the only inference to be drawn from this example it is
especially noteworthy if the person has a known history
of previous depressive episodes requiring admission to
hospital.

A negative attitude to admission may be inferred from
the behaviour of an underweight teenage girl almost as
soon as she and her mother arrive at the unit. From the
absence of any mother–daughter interaction the conclu-
sion may be drawn that the girl's resentment at being in
hospital is related to her mother's insistence that professional help be sought: the girl may wish to continue her
relentless pursuit of thinness.

As well as making subjective inferences and interpretations the nurse uses objective observations during the
assessment process. She will note the person's rate and
content of speech, ability to concentrate and willingness
to respond to questions, and the amount of eye
contact—if any—during the interview. Non-verbal cues

such as facial expression, posture and degree of activity are also noted. From time to time observation of the person's physical condition gives rise for concern and may require immediate attention.

All observation is selective, however, and it is important to be aware of the way expectations, attention, preoccupations and prior knowledge affect what is observed. It may therefore be useful to compare observations with those of other nurses, noting where these conflict, and to try to identify possible reasons for these variations.

Cultural differences in behaviour. A knowledge of normal behavioural patterns in different cultural groups is essential if an accurate assessment of the patient is to be made. What is accepted as normal behaviour differs with social, educational and ethnic background. It is important to observe to what extent patients' behaviour deviates from that accepted by their own group. Without a knowledge of sociology there is a danger that the nurse's own social and educational background may bias observations. Where nurses and patients come from different ethnic backgrounds, particularly if they do not share a language, special care is needed to make observations valid.

Abnormal behaviour in psychiatric disorders. The nurse should be acquainted with patterns of abnormal behaviour and their incidence in various psychiatric disorders (see Appendix A). A knowledge of psychology and of psychiatric illness may help to detect the earliest manifestations of disorder, when these may well be atypical and different in each patient. But it is very important to be aware of the effect of 'labelling' a patient. Once a patient has a diagnostic label attached, for example schizophrenia, the nurse may believe she observes symptoms which in reality are not there. An illustration of distorted perceptions by members of the nursing staff can be found in the much-quoted and disturbing account by Rosenham (1973) of the experiences of a group of pseudopatients in the USA. These people allegedly heard 'voices' and were all, with only one exception, given a diagnosis of schizophrenia. The diagnosis persisted throughout their stay in hospital notwithstanding the fact that on admission they gave up any pretence of mental disorder and behaved normally. Ironically their fellow patients were not deceived; they quickly realized that the 'patients' were perfectly normal individuals, in hospital under false pretences, whereas the nursing staff repeatedly 'observed' their behaviour to be consistent with the label of schizophrenia.

Participant observation and observer effect. The nurse should be with the patient for sufficient time to be able to report on the total picture presented. Only if she knows him well can she observe minor variations in behaviour.

The nurse should not disturb the patient by her presence. This means that she must be in the ward so much that her presence is taken for granted and that she is sufficiently unobtrusive for patients to behave as if she were not there at all. It is easiest to observe the patient's behaviour if one joins in all the activities. If the nurse supervises passively, doing nothing while the patient is expected to take part in some ward activity, her presence may be resented and the impression she gains then becomes distorted. If she comes and goes, she disturbs the patient's activities and cannot really observe.

Objectivity. The distinction was drawn earlier between subjectivity in the assessment process—using inferences and interpretations—and objective observations from observable behaviour. Objectivity, while more scientific than subjectivity, is not always entirely possible, though structured forms and rating scales, specially designed as assessment tools, do help (see above). It is important that the nurse does not allow herself to become disturbed or shocked by the patient's behaviour. Her interest in the patient's recovery should not make her emotionally biased (see p. 100). She should not feel flattered at, or proud of, the patient's improvement, since this might lead her to see improvements where there are none. One of the reasons why relatives are sometimes unreliable informants is their inability to remain objective.

Bias and selectivity. The nurse should remember to observe not only the patient, but the situation in which the patient finds himself. To do this is relatively easy when the nurse's observation concerns the interaction between several patients, or that between the patient and another nurse. It is much more difficult if the nurse is observing an incident in which she herself has participated. The patient's behaviour which she observes may then be a reaction to her words, actions or gestures. It may require considerable mental effort to report such behaviour not as it appeared to her, but as she imagines it might have appeared to a third person. Her own part in the interaction needs to be reported as well as the patient's.

Recording and reporting observations. As noted earlier, it is impossible to observe the patient's behaviour without to some extent drawing inferences and forming conclusions, but it is essential that observed facts be reported, and not merely opinions; or at least that, when opinions are given, these should provide some indication of the facts on which they are based. It is important for the nurse to remember that nursing records might have to be produced in court at some time in the future; therefore accuracy in documenting facts is essential.

Clichés should, as far as possible, be avoided. Such words as 'pleasant and cooperative' mean nothing unless it is stated who finds the patient pleasant and for what reason, and what were the tasks in which the patient was expected to cooperate. 'Uncooperative', again, describes the relationship between the patient and someone else. It is important to know with whom the patient refused to cooperate, and what attempts were made to persuade him or her to do so.

Some expressions, such as 'bizarre behaviour' or 'incoherent speech', are meaningful to a certain extent, because they are used by most people to apply to the same kinds of phenomena. Nevertheless, definite examples are better than the mere statement that the nurse failed to understand the patient.

After a thorough assessment of the needs of the person who requires professional help the nurse can then proceed to the second stage of the nursing process.

2   Planning Care

The nursing activities involved in this stage of the nursing process include:

- setting clear goals;
- compiling a written care plan;
- involving clients' participation.

Advantages of goal setting. Identifying specific goals provides a valuable opportunity to guide the nursing interventions required to meet clients' needs. Goal setting also assists in the evaluation of both clients' progress and the effectiveness of the care.

Setting goals which are time-limited, and documented as either of short- medium- or long-term duration, helps focus the activities of the nursing team. Goals must be realistic and agreed with the client. In a rehabilitation unit, for example, early success in achieving a realistic short-term goal can be most encouraging for a person with enduring mental health problems and provides the motivation to proceed with his rehabilitation programme: failure to achieve an unrealistic goal is demoralizing and demotivating (Ironbar & Hooper, 1989).

Nursing care plans. Care planning involves the use of written nursing care plans for recording details of the care to be given and of its evaluation at some later specified date. They are formulated by the primary nurse/key worker in discussion with the client, relatives and other members of the multidisciplinary care team. Care plans differ widely in their design: the example shown in Figure 4.1 gives basic information of clients' needs, goals, nursing actions and evaluation of care.

Client involvement in planning care. An integral part of the above activities is the active involvement of the client as a collaborative partner with the nursing team—whenever possible—in the planning of his care.

Many people appreciate the opportunity afforded for empowerment through participation in the planning of their own care but careful thought is also given to those for whom this may be neither appropriate nor wholly desirable.

A modification to client's participation is required, however, when goals for safety needs are being identified. For example, some severely depressed people's

Needs	Goals	Nursing actions	Evaluation (daily)
To have delusional talk responded to appropriately	To convey empathy through communication After nurse's response Mrs K will be able to engage in a simple diversional activity	Respond to feeling tone rather than content Indicate appreciation of distress Give honest account of origin of Mrs K's thoughts Do not reinforce or argue with Mrs K	By observing that Mrs K appears less distressed in the presence of her key worker By observing the period of time Mrs K spends on an activity without expressing delusional ideas

Fig. 4.1 Mrs K's care plan.

goal is to try to harm themselves whereas that of the nursing team is to prevent this from happening by 'constant observation' (see below). While this particular planning decision has to be taken unilaterally by the nursing (and medical) team, other aspects of such clients' care can still be planned with their active involvement.

Linked to planning care for clients' safety needs is the practice in many acute psychiatric units of having a written hospital policy which ensures that each person on admission is individually assigned to a category indicating the level of supervision (observation) required. A note of the agreed category is recorded in the person's medical notes and nursing plans.

Maximum supervision. A person who is transferred from intensive care after emergency treatment for a suicidal attempt is likely, for example, to be classified as requiring maximum supervision (also known as constant observation or 'specialling'); this means one-to-one client–nurse contact throughout day and night.

Close observation. Clients classified as being at a moderately high risk of harming themselves may require close observation by nursing staff. Gardner (1991) recommends that this person is 'seen by the nursing staff at least once in every 10 minutes' during the day and is also observed at frequent intervals by night staff. As the person improves so the intervals between checks lengthen. There is considerable variation in levels of supervision categories among hospitals and learners should find out exactly what is expected of them.

Standard observation. People who are not considered at risk may only need to report to the nurse in charge before leaving the unit for any reason, say where they are going, with whom and when they hope to return.

Use of care plans for research. An important reason for keeping a detailed written record of the care plan (and the nursing care given) is that detailed records can be used later for research purposes. It may be difficult to be sure that actions have had the desired effect on an individual patient, but to collect in retrospect evidence of what has been done on a number of occasions by different nurses and with many patients is an important step in developing a distinctive nursing practice.

Well-documented nursing care plans and accurate progress reports help immeasurably in coordinating teamwork. It is of interest to compare the perspective brought to bear on any one patient's care by different members of the multidisciplinary care team.

A final reason for detailed individualized care plans lies in *the nature of psychiatric care.* Much of what goes on in a ward setting affects all, or at least many, patients simultaneously. A community meeting may concern itself with a problem to several patients; an accident to one patient on the ward affects all; so does the admission of new patients, a patient's death or an episode of disturbed behaviour. *How* specifically an event affects a particular patient needs to be recorded by his or her primary nurse who may also have to adapt the subsequent care plan in the light of the way the patient was able to cope.

3 Implementation or Delivery of the Planned Care

The third stage of the nursing process is implementation and this encompasses the delivery of the appropriate nursing interventions agreed with the patient in the planning process in order to achieve the goals detailed in the plan of care. In Section III of this book some specific examples of nursing interventions are described. Without this stage of the nursing process, and the last, evaluation, the first and second stages would be meaningless, academic exercises.

4 Evaluation of the Care Given

Although it is essential to have some criteria by which to evaluate the care which has been given to an individual it is in practice very difficult to isolate the effect of any one part of what happens to patients from the others. To evaluate care accurately it is necessary to know not only what nurses and other team members have been doing but also what the influence of other patients or the patient's relatives and friends has been.

Self-assessment by the patient, using a rating scale, may be one criterion of value to evaluate progress over a

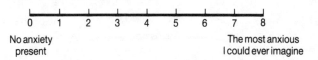

Fig. 4.2 An 8-point rating scale.

period of several weeks or months. An 8-point scale may be filled in by a person who has high anxiety levels, before, during and after exposure to the feared object or situation (Figure 4.2). If the therapy is successful, the degree of anxiety experienced ought to decrease over time; the scales represent a written record and evaluation of the improvement. Another example cited by Ritter (1989) is a 10-point rating scale on which the person is asked to record the progress he feels he has made towards reaching his goals (Figure 4.3).

A depression inventory, completed by a depressed person before and after therapeutic interventions, and questionnaires, filled in by someone who, for example, has been learning to adopt new anxiety management techniques, are also useful evaluation tools.

Evaluation by the nursing staff will be happening all the time and every day, but a specific date and time needs to be set aside for a thorough look at what has been achieved, what still needs to be done, what is the best way of proceeding, what has worked in the past or what has not been helpful. New goals or targets are set and the process continues until the patient has recovered, is ready to be discharged home, or requires further care involving people outside hospital. This then becomes the

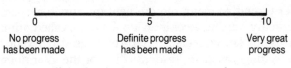

Fig. 4.3 A 10-point progress scale.

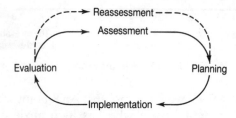

Fig. 4.4   The spiral nature of the nursing process.

responsibility of the Community Mental Health Team, some of whom may be the same members of the hospital multidisciplinary team but who continue to work with people who are living in the community outside hospital.

The nursing process is, therefore, a continuing process leading from *assessment* to *planning* to *implementation* to *evaluation* to *reassessment* and so on (Figure 4.4).

PRIMARY NURSING

The second of the three innovations in nursing practice to be described in this chapter is the organization and delivery of care known as *primary nursing*. It was first described in detail by Manthey *et al.* (1970) in the US and is now firmly established practice in a number of clinical settings in this country. Much of the pioneering work in the UK has been carried out in nursing development units (NDUs), i.e. units which admit people—often elderly—with a major requirement for nursing.

Primary nursing gives individual nurses, called primary nurses, (or 'key workers', the term often used in psychiatric care settings) primary responsibility for the total nursing care of an assigned group of patients, numbering from three to six usually, throughout their stay in hospital. This nurse has *continuous* responsibility for the planning and delivery of care, 24 hours of the day, seven days a week. An associate nurse deputizes for the primary nurse when the latter is off duty and may make changes to the care plan to reflect changes in the patient's condition. Nevertheless, it is the primary nurse who has the ultimate responsibility for any major changes in the overall design of the plan.

Additionally the primary nurse is accountable for the standard of care she gives to the individuals in her group. She is also accountable to the person's family, to her nursing colleagues and to other members of the multidisciplinary team for the care she delivers.

Primary nursing is especially suited to the practice of psychiatric and mental health nursing, irrespective of the care setting, facilitating as it does frequent one-to-one nurse–patient interactions. Evaluating primary nursing McMahon (1990) comments that there is an important underlying assumption in this method of organizing and delivering nursing care that the nurse–patient relationship is a valuable ingredient for success, the primary nurse being ideally placed to get 'close' to the individuals in her care, allowing her to work in partnership with them.

Continuity and consistency of care are other advantages offered by primary nursing to the person with a psychiatric disorder. These benefits are highlighted by Ritter (1985) in a description of the care of a severely depressed woman. Examining this patient's past records from another hospital Ritter identified the handwriting of 12 different nurses who had been caring for her during the first eight weeks of her stay in hospital. The introduction of primary nursing spared this woman the feelings of rejection sometimes experienced by those whose care is delivered by a large number of nurses and who may as a result be subjected to many different policies.

A research project by Armitage (1988) examines the implementation of primary nursing in two long-stay psychiatric wards. A brief account of some of his findings is given in a later chapter (see p. 192).

The Key Worker in Day Hospitals

Attenders at day hospitals also benefit enormously from having an identifiable key worker who is accountable for discussing details of their care programme/plan with them on a regular basis. However, to prevent the client from becoming overdependent on one person, and in turn to avoid undue pressure on the key worker, parts of the care may be shared with another member of the day hospital's multidisciplinary team.

The use of the term key worker is not confined to a nurse practitioner: the key worker for certain clients residing in the community could be a community psychiatric nurse but equally might be a social worker or an occupational therapist—an identified person who is responsible for coordinating clients' care.

MODELS OF CARE

In the recent past much of mental health and psychiatric nursing care has been dominated by non-nursing models. For example:

- the *medical model* with its emphasis on diagnoses and medical treatments, and
- the *behavioural model*, introduced by clinical psychologists and focusing on techniques designed to change maladaptive behaviour.

Few nurse practitioners would wish to deny that the theories underpinning non-nursing models have relevance for their work but rightly assert only a model of nursing can provide the framework necessary to identify specifically nursing needs and inform nursing actions.

Evidence of a movement away from dependence on non-nursing models towards the development of psychiatric nursing as a discipline in its own right is increasingly being found. Nurses are taking charge of their own professional skills, knowledge and expertise, irrespective of their area of work, and beginning to function as equal partners in the multidisciplinary team. As stated earlier in this chapter, this heightening of nursing's profile, together (it is hoped) with improvements in patient care, has been facilitated by the changes in the organization of care effected by the nursing process and primary nursing and, more recently, with the use of models of nursing.

Models of Nursing Care

A model of nursing may be defined as a framework which can be used as a guideline for the assessment, identification of an individual's needs, the planning and implementation required to meet these needs and the evaluation of the effectiveness of the nursing actions.

According to Minshull *et al*. (1986) 'problems have arisen because nurses frequently have not had an overt model of nursing from which to develop a framework for assessment'.

Around 40 nursing models have been formulated by nurse academics and most bear the name of their creators. All are based on a theory or group of theories and are sometimes referred to as 'theoretical models' (Reynolds & Cormack, 1990).

Four models of nursing in use in psychiatric nursing are included in this chapter.

- Orem's Self-care Model
- Peplau's Interpersonal Model
- Activities of Living Model
- The Human Needs Model

Orem's Self-care Model

The self-care model is mentioned first because of its importance in the trend discussed earlier towards the development of an independent practice of nursing and the recognition of the uniqueness of the contribution of the nurse. In the application of this model to psychiatric nursing, the individual's psychiatric disorder and consequent psychological problems are not ignored but seen in the light of their effects on the individual's self-care difficulties. As a result the primary focus for the initiation of nursing interventions is the person's inability to engage in an area of self-care rather than on the fact that he suffers, for example, from the negative symptoms of schizophrenia.

Self-care is defined by Orem (1985) as '. . . the practice of activities that individuals initiate to perform on their own behalf in maintenance of life, health and well being'. Although Orem's ideas largely originate from her own experiences she does acknowledge the work of other nurse theorists and social scientists; two examples of theoretical concepts she uses to underpin her model—the self-care deficit and the nursing systems theories—are outlined in this section.

Self-care Deficit Theory

A self-care deficit exists when a person's self-care ability is less than his self-care demands. In order to identify a person's self-care deficits assessment data are usually categorized under three headings: universal, developmental and health deviation.

Universal. Concerned with a person's ability to carry out the daily living skills required to maintain physical, mental and social well-being.

Developmental. Associated with mental and physical lifespan development. Assessment is made of an individual's ability to cope with crises and life events arising from developmental or environmental causes. Additionally account is taken of any repercussions such events may have on overall self-care demands. A recently bereaved person, for example, may be unable to meet the 'universal' self-care demand to sleep a specific number of hours each night.

Health deviation. This relates to a person's ability to manage the effects of illness or injury, such as being able to comply with drug treatment and to recognize the possibility of unwanted side-effects. Assessment will also include a person's ability to make satisfactory adjustment to a chronic disability or to come to terms with an alteration in body image resulting from say surgical intervention or a neurological deficit. Failure to adapt may have contributed to a person's current mental health problems.

Nursing Systems Theory

This theory explains the therapeutic nature of the nursing interventions planned to assist the person—and his family where applicable—to achieve self-care. These interventions may be implemented in one of three ways:

1   *The wholly compensatory nursing system.* In this nursing situation the patient performs little or no active role in his care. An example may be the very severely depressed person who is unable to meet any of the self-care demands without prompting or assistance from the nurse.

2   *The partly compensatory system.* This system describes a situation in which the nurse and patient are both active partners in care. Such a situation might obtain in a rehabilitation unit when the resident first embarks on a structured programme of activities geared towards eventual discharge.

3   *The supportive–educative system.* In this nursing system the nurse is required only to offer support and encouragement as the patient becomes proficient in, say, decision-making skills; she may also be available in a consultative capacity as and when necessary.
   It will be noted that this last-mentioned system, which focuses on the helping role of maximizing a person's self-care abilities through education, guidance and psychological support, closely corresponds to the work of the CPN—as described in Chapter 3—and accounts for the growing popularity of Orem's model in community care.

Peplau's Interpersonal Model

This model has as its main theme the development of the therapeutic relationship between patient and nurse. Categorized as a developmental model of nursing, Peplau's is one of the most important and best known in psychiatric and mental health nursing circles. Peplau (1952) states that nursing is a 'significant therapeutic interpersonal process which functions cooperatively with other human processes that make health possible for individuals', and as with Orem's her model emphatically endorses the distinctive role of nursing practice.

The theory underpinning Peplau's interpersonal model stresses that for a successful relationship to develop the nurse must always be aware of the effect her responses have on the patient and be able to learn from these interactions.

Peplau's theory also explores the tensions associated with anxiety which arise when the drive for security (both psychological and physical) within the individual is frustrated. The care required to alleviate this person's anxiety is described in four phases similar to—though anticipating by several years—the nursing process.

The four stages briefly described are:

1 *Orientation phase.* This may be linked to the assessment stage of the nursing process. This stage allows for information to be gathered while at the same time providing an opportunity for the individual to get to know the nurse and vice versa.

2 *Identification phase.* During this phase a plan is negotiated and the nurse sets goals after the person has had the opportunity to express his feelings. It is the nurse's responsibility to set these goals. (See p. 57 for an example of the severely depressed patient whose own

goals may be detrimental to his safety and will differ from those of the nurse.)

3   *Exploitation*. This third phase is concerned with the measures taken by the nurse to help relieve the patient's anxieties. Peplau's concept of the 'nearness of the nurse' is highlighted in this phase of the development of the relationship. Help may also be enlisted from other members of the multidisciplinary care team at this point.

4   *Resolution*. Finally, as the name suggests, many if not all of the patient's difficulties have been resolved at this stage. The patient may reflect on the growth and development in self-understanding which has taken place and on how he will be able to cope should similar difficulties re-emerge in future. The nurse for her part will have progressed considerably in her ability to respond appropriately when caring for subsequent patients.

Practical application of some aspects of Peplau's model of nursing care may be found in Chapter 6.

Activities of Living Model

Roper, Logan and Tierney's Activities of Living Model (Roper *et al.*, 1990), is British-born unlike most of the other nursing models currently in use in the UK.

Roper and her colleagues emphasize the need for nurses to focus their attention on the patient's *observable* and *measurable behaviours*, rather than, as formerly, placing reliance solely on, say, intuition when giving care.

This model has been categorized as an example of a behavioural model because its theoretical base stems from the behavioural school of psychology with its commitment to the scientific rigour required for the accurate observation and measurement of behaviour. The creators of this model of nursing also recognize that assessment is the foundation of the nursing process and regard their model as a useful basic framework to assess specific patient behaviours known as activities of living. Roper, Logan and Tierney assert that humans engage in 12 activities of living in the course of their lifespan, from birth to death, which is a continuum on which their degree of dependence or independence varies, influenced by changes in the physical, psychological, social, cultural or economic environment in which they are at any one time.

The activities of living are listed below—the first *seven* are regarded as essential for the maintenance of life (Roper *et al.*, 1990).

1 Maintaining a safe environment
2 Breathing
3 Eating and drinking
4 Eliminating
5 Controlling body temperature
6 Mobilizing
7 Sleeping
8 Communicating
9 Personal cleansing and dressing
10 Working and playing
11 Expressing sexuality
12 Dying

These seven activities of living based on the physical needs of the patient explain the value of this model in the care of the person whose physical needs predominate; it has been included in this chapter because of its almost 'blanket implementation' in the UK (Walsh, 1991). Roper's model is of limited use in psychiatric settings but selected areas may be 'borrowed' when assessing the physical needs of, for example, the elated and overactive person who is too 'busy' to attend to such mundane matters.

Choosing a Model of Nursing

Currently there are some forty or so models available. Regardless of the care setting, the difficult decision faced by practitioners when selecting one of the forty may be influenced by their personal beliefs and values (philosophy) on what nursing should be about.

It is our opinion that the model of nursing chosen should reflect a philosophy based on a commitment to the holistic approach to care, that is the relatively recent acceptance by the nursing profession of the need to take cognizance of the total functioning of the person and of the interdependency of his psychological, physical, social and spiritual needs.

Orem's model of nursing—the first to be described in this chapter—has a firm commitment to the concept that the individual is to be cared for as a whole person, but Minshull *et al.* (1986), while acknowledging that the work of Orem cannot be ignored, comment that they were unable to find a nursing model which met *all* their criteria—one of which was that equal emphasis be placed on all aspects of human needs—and created their own. It is known as 'the human needs model of nursing': the fourth model to be discussed in this section.

This is a model adapted from the humanist psychologist Maslow's motivational theory of human needs (Maslow, 1954). The humanists expounded their theories of psychology after the behaviourists and they criticized their predecessors for concentrating exclusively on behaviour; of taking too narrow and simplistic a view of the nature of human beings.

Maslow arranged human needs in a hierarchical triangle (Figure 4.5). Lower needs, such as physical, safety and security, were placed near its base; higher needs, for example love, belonging, dignity and self-esteem, came above them.

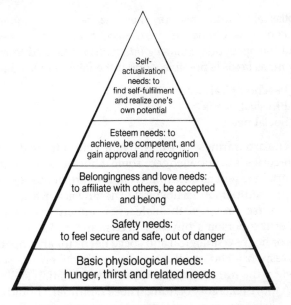

Fig. 4.5 Maslow's hierarchy of needs.

This hierarchy of needs has practical application in psychiatric and mental health nursing care: physical and safety needs of the severely depressed patient, if unmet, could endanger his life and require to be assessed on admission before his less urgent, though no less important, psychological needs.

The human needs model of nursing reflects our beliefs and values, outlined earlier; they are reiterated by Minshull and her colleagues: 'the individual within this model is viewed holistically, having interdependent physical, psychological, spiritual and social needs'.

In the next section of this book, devoted to nursing care of people in a variety of settings, an adaptation of the human needs model is used. Each individual is viewed holistically and his or her needs are frequently categorized—often related to the *identification* of these needs and the appropriate *nursing interventions* required to meet them, as far as is possible—under the following headings.

- Psychological needs
- Physical needs
- Social needs

The arbitrariness of this separation into three discrete categories is acknowledged: some if not all can overlap to a certain extent as exemplified in the care of the severely depressed person in hospital. The physical presence of the nurse provides the safe environment required to meet the person's physical needs, and simultaneously his or her psychological and social needs for an empathetic response and social interaction respectively are being met by the nurse's expertise in communication skills.

A fourth category of human need, spiritual, should also be considered if a holistic approach to care is used. To try to satisfy the needs of those clients who have a religious faith it is necessary for nurses to be fully conversant with the pastoral care available in their place of work.

Initially on admission, for example, basic factual information such as the person's religious status is usually elicited; later as a result of nurses' 24 hour contact with clients, they are uniquely placed to assess any such needs and to liaise—if the person so wishes—with the appropriate religious representative. In the meantime, the person may be comforted by having the opportunity to talk over feelings with a nurse who is prepared to listen attentively and to respond in a sensitive and supportive manner. A similar response from a nurse may be appreciated by the person who has no particular religious belief but might equally like the opportunity to give expression to his or her individual spiritual needs.

SUMMARY

This chapter has briefly discussed three methods currently in use in relation to the organization and delivery of nursing care: the nursing process, primary nursing and models of nursing. Such important developments in nursing practice have collectively effected an enhancement in the quality of patient care and have led to a heightened awareness of the uniqueness and significance of the role of the nurse in the multidisciplinary care team. Additionally they have substantially strengthened nursing's theoretical base without which practice might have remained at best intuitive and empathic, at worst lacking in any underlying rationale for care.

FURTHER READING

Aggleton P & Chalmers H (1992) Peplau's development model. *Nursing Times* **86**(2): 38–40.

Cavanagh S (1991) Orem and the Nursing Process. New directions for the 90s. *Nursing Practice* **4**: 26.

Macdonald M (1988) Primary nursing: is it worth it? *Journal of Advanced Nursing* **13**: 797–806.

Moores A (1987) Facing the fear. *Nursing Times* **83**(27): 44–46.

Pearson A (1988) *Primary Nursing: Nursing in the Burford and Oxford Development Units*: London: Croom Helm.

Salvage J (1990) The theory and practice of the 'new nursing'. *Nursing Times Occasional Paper* **86**(1): 42–45.

Underwood P & Meuser S (1990) Orem's self-care model: clinical applications. In: Reynolds W & Cormack D (eds) *Psychiatric and Mental Health Nursing*. London: Chapman & Hall.

Wesley R (1992) *Nursing Theories and Models*. Pennsylvania: Springfield Corporation.

REFERENCES

Armitage P (1988) Changing care: an evaluation of primary nursing in psychiatric long-term care. Unpublished report School of Nursing Studies, University of Wales College of Medicine, Cardiff.

Barker P (1986) *Assessment in Psychiatric Nursing*. London: Croom Helm.

Brooker C & Baguley I (1990) SNAP decisions. *Nursing Times* **86**(41): 56–58.

Gardner R (1991) *Guidelines on the Clinical Management of Suicidal Patients in Hospital*. Cambridge Mental Health Services.

Ironbar O & Hooper A (1989) *Self-instruction in Mental Health Nursing*. London: Baillière Tindall.

Manthey M, Ciske K, Robertson P *et al.* (1970) *Primary Nursing Forum* **9**(i): 64–83.

Maslow A (1954) *Motivation and Personality*. London: Harper & Row.

McMahon R (1990) Collegiality is the key. *Nursing Times* **86**(42): 66–67.

Minshull J, Ross K & Turner J (1986) The human needs model of nursing. *Journal of Advanced Nursing* **11**: 643–649.

Mulhearn S (1989) The nursing process: improving psychiatric admission assessment. *Journal of Advanced Nursing* **14**: 808–813.

Orem D (1985) *Nursing: Concepts of Practice*. New York: McGraw-Hill.

Peplau H (1952) *Interpersonal Relations in Nursing*. New York: Putman.

Reynolds W & Cormack D (1990) *Psychiatric and Mental Health Nursing*. London: Chapman & Hall.

Ritter S (1985) Primary nursing in mental illness. *Nursing Mirror* **160**(17): 16.

Ritter S (1989) *Manual of Clinical Psychiatric Nursing: Principles and Procedures*. London: Harper & Row.

Roper N, Logan W & Tierney A (1990) *The Elements of Nursing*. Edinburgh: Churchill Livingstone.

Rosenham D (1973) On being sane in insane places. *Science* **1179**: 250–258.

Tissier J (1986) The development of a psychiatric nursing assessment form. In: Brooking J (ed.) *Psychiatric Nursing Research*. Chichester: Wiley.

Walsh M (1991) *Models in Clinical Nursing: The Way Forward*. London: Baillière Tindall.

SECTION III: CARING FOR PEOPLE IN A VARIETY OF SETTINGS

Chapter 5
Admission to Hospital

INTRODUCTION

Before admission to hospital people have often lived through a period of considerable tension and strain. People with mental health problems may have realized their increasing inability to adjust to the demands made on them and after desperate attempts to cope may have broken down suddenly under the stress, or may gradually have understood the need for professional help. The individual's family may also have been exposed to a great deal of strain. Often as a person's symptoms develop they are subjected to comment, criticism and reproach. Gradually, however, the relatives realize the sufferer is unable to do anything about how he or she feels and behaves, and become worried and anxious. As the need for admission to hospital becomes obvious and imminent, they start to feel guilty and partially responsible for their loved one's condition, ashamed and emotionally drained.

Added to feelings of guilt, are misconceptions about psychiatric hospitals that may occasionally—even today—cause the family to delay as long as possible their relative's admission. In almost every case, and particularly if compulsory legal measures have to be taken (see

Appendix B), or considerable effort expended in persuading the person to accept help, admission to a psychiatric hospital represents a crisis in the individual's life and that of his or her family; it can mark the climax of an intensely distressing home situation.

ADMISSION TO HOSPITAL

Most people are apprehensive at the thought of having to be admitted to hospital, but these feelings are exacerbated when admission to a psychiatric hospital is necessary. Reasons for feeling anxious are varied. For example, some people are

- acutely aware of adverse media coverage;
- afraid that once in hospital their stay will be prolonged;
- worried about the stigma attached to psychiatric hospitals;
- convinced that their loved ones, friends and colleagues will think less of them for having been in a psychiatric hospital.

Other individuals have feelings of inadequacy and guilt and are certain that mental health is purely a matter of will power, despite their family doctor's protestations that this is not so; they may despise themselves for having 'given-in' instead of 'pulling themselves together' and overcoming their difficulties without help.

Nurses therefore have an essential role to play in helping to gradually reduce the high levels of anxiety experienced by most newcomers to a psychiatric unit. In order to achieve this goal, it is important that staff are able to convey warmth and friendliness, and to show genuine appreciation of the underlying reasons for the person's anxieties.

Nevertheless, despite the nursing staff's determined efforts to create a welcoming and relaxed atmosphere, newcomers can still feel very bewildered, embarrassed and insecure as a result of the many new experiences of admission. Though they may wish to ask many questions they may feel unable to give voice to any of them at first. The nurse's positive and concerned attitude can encourage new clients to talk about their fears and to admit to any misconceptions they may have. What is very much appreciated by newly admitted clients is a nurse who is approachable and willing to listen attentively in an unhurried manner to what is being said and whose responses suggest a desire to try to find out and to understand more about what is worrying the person.

Nothing the person wants to know is too trivial for discussion, but he or she cannot always formulate or articulate problems clearly. In the early days following admission, answers to clients' questions may not in fact be known, but that should not prevent the person from asking. Whenever an answer is possible it should be frank and straightforward. But hasty answers, before questions are fully expressed, merely serve to convince the person of the futility of asking.

Conversely the answer to the important question of confidentiality should be answered by the nurse before the client needs to ask: it can be a great relief to know that all information given is considered as being strictly confidential, that nothing will be disclosed to anyone other than those members of the multidisciplinary care team who are directly involved in their care.

Some of the words and actions of disturbed people are capable of causing considerable embarrassment at a later date (see Chapter 8) and they must be able to rely implicitly on the integrity of every member of the care team to observe complete confidentiality.

SUMMARY

People entering a psychiatric hospital have anxieties and fears of a different nature from those who are admitted for a physical disorder. The sensitive and concerned nurse who is aware of the newly admitted person's anxieties can help by being available to listen and to give considered and informed replies to questions. It is reassuring for the client to know that any information disclosed is passed only to those directly responsible for his or her care.

Chapter 6
Human Interactions and Relationships

INTRODUCTION

This chapter examines in some detail the *universal and crucial need* of the person with mental health problems for communication, both verbal and non-verbal. In trying to satisfy this need, the nursing staff require to take part in *interactions* with the patient so that a helping *relationship* may be established.

Later chapters will look at some of the *specific needs* and nursing interventions when caring for people in a variety of settings.

HUMAN INTERACTIONS

Patients' Reactions to Hospital Admission

During the first few days in hospital (or in any new setting) the individual is among strangers. He naturally feels insecure and diffident. His attitude to the people who are concerned with his care is affected by this. Some people show their anxiety, others appear full of self-confidence or even a little brash or aggressive. Later the person's behaviour may be very different from the initial impression he created. It is important to take his first approach seriously, as his attitude may be characteristic of the way he behaves towards strangers. Shyness or diffidence or apparent aggressiveness may be part of the difficulty in meeting people.

The preliminary period of getting to know one another is a very important phase in establishing confidence. No-one is quite free from preconceived ideas. 'Hospital', 'psychiatric hospital', 'day hospital', 'day centre', 'nurse', 'community psychiatric nurse', are all words which conjure up mental pictures for everybody, pictures which often correspond very little to reality and are determined by past experience and by some ideal which is popularly accepted.

The person's ready-made attitude to nurses may be important in helping him to accept his new situation. To many people the title 'nurse' stands for all that is good, kind and competent. This stereotype is, of course, quite unrealistic; nurses are only human, each nurse is different and no nurse embodies all the good qualities which people expect in the ideal nurse. Nevertheless, the fact that people tend to be well disposed to nurses and to trust them may help reduce some of their initial anxiety.

Introductions are important in that they stress the nurse's personality rather than her role. The person is often more interested in her name than in her rank in the nursing hierarchy. Although the use of first names is widespread in psychiatric care settings each individual is given the opportunity to state his or her preference. Some people feel uncomfortable if they are addressed by the name normally used only by members of their immediate family or close friends (Dobbin, 1990).

Initial Patient–Nurse Interactions

Conversational Topics

The process of becoming acquainted is a mutual one. While the nurse tries to find out as much as possible about the person in order to help him, the person tries to find out as much as possible about the nurses in order to establish which ones have authority and/or can be trusted. Only when he becomes convinced that a nurse genuinely feels interested in him and does not criticize him, does he continue to single her out and give her an opportunity of learning more about him. Every time the nurse converses with the individual, alone or in a group, she acquires more information about him.

Conversation with the patient rarely touches on personal problems in the early stages. It may not be wise for the nurse to ask direct questions. The aim of this initial talking with the patient is not primarily to find out about his disorder but to get to know him as a person. Anything that interests him is a good starting point—sport, his (or her) work, a television programme or the contents of the newspaper. Gradually it becomes possible to build up a picture of the way the person spent his (or her) life before seeking professional help.

Discussion of the newspapers not only has the value of keeping people informed and up to date but also touches on many opinions. Politics and religion are topics which cannot really be avoided, though some nurses endeavour to do so. These subjects are so important in most people's lives that any conversation attempting to circumvent them becomes artificial. There is no harm in hearing the patient's views or in stimulating him to further thought. These subjects only become difficult if the nurse's own views are so dogmatic, or if she is so emotional about them, that she cannot listen calmly to the patient. It is also important that the patient should feel completely free from pressure and that he should never come to think that his treatment might be jeopardized by the fact that his political or religious convictions are not those of a particular member of staff.

Learning More About Each Other

Most conversations, however apparently neutral the topic, tend to reveal some of the patient's specific difficulties. Although the nurse may not have asked a question, she may soon become aware that the patient's political opinions have a delusional quality or that the topic of the educational system of the country is one about which husband and wife disagree, or that, although the patient's mother lives nearby, she never visits. It is much better for information to be pieced together gradually than to press the patient for personal details.

While the nurse gets to know the patient, the patient learns a great deal about the nurse. Every occasion when nurse and patient are together offers as much opportunity to the patient as it does to the nurse. The nurse's tact, the genuineness of her interest are among the personal characteristics the patient notices. Gestures, facial expression, tone of voice sometimes convey much more than actual words. A patient can usually judge if the nurse enjoys spending time with him or is merely doing so from a sense of duty.

Patients often remember what was talked about on the last occasion and if the nurse forgets, it is interpreted as a clear sign that she could not have been very interested; this may be disappointing or even insulting to the patient. By contrast, to refer back to something the patient mentioned last time or to ask him about his activities on the day the nurse was off duty indicates interest.

A patient not only judges the nurse's behaviour to him personally but also takes into account her behaviour to others. It is comforting to see another seriously disturbed patient competently and kindly dealt with and extremely worrying to see a nurse ignore someone in need of help or deal hastily with another patient. Each patient feels that the treatment meted out to another might easily happen to him.

Each patient's personal needs also determine the way in which he sees and uses the staff. A patient may find someone whose interest and concern he values and whom he dislikes at the same time for making him dependent on her. Another patient, feeling weak and insecure, develops a growing attachment to a nurse whose forceful personality he needs, while yet another treats the same nurse with hostility, rudeness and scorn, because he sees in her a representative authority and he treats authority with his usual defiance and resentment. The patient's attitude to any one nurse may change during his stay in hospital, sometimes rapidly, sometimes over a period of time. It is usually interesting and worthwhile trying to find out what has caused changes in relationships, but this is not always possible to establish. Something in the nurse's tone of voice, her facial expression or her manner, may have conveyed to the patient disapproval or criticism, even if none was intended. Some reaction may not have been in keeping with the role which for the time being the nurse has fulfilled towards the patient. The patient may have expected protection and found that the nurse expected him to manage without it. He may have hoped for disapproval, but found the nurse non-committal. He may have expected affection and have felt rejected.

The ease with which nurse and patient interact depends to a large extent on the personal characteristics of the people concerned. Patients and nurses with similar interests and backgrounds may find it easy to talk to one another. The patient's age also plays a part in interactions. Some nurses find older patients easier to talk to than patients of their own age, others find the reverse to be true.

Not all interactions between nurses and patients exert an influence on the patient's recovery, especially when the nurse's allocation to a unit is of short duration. Many interactions merely serve to make the patient's stay more interesting, to reduce boredom or to convey to the patient a general sense of concern and interest in his welfare. A few, however, can make important contributions to the patient's progress. These occur from the nurse's sensitive appreciation of the patient's mood, preoccupation and thought, gained during regular contact with him. Unless frequent interactions occur, the opportunity for extended contact will be missed.

Therapeutic Interactions

Taking Account of the Patient's Emotional State

The patient's emotional state affects the extent to which he chooses or is able to interact with nurses, and also the extent to which some nurses choose to interact with patients (Altschul, 1972).

A person distressed, for example, about 'voices' (i.e. auditory hallucinations—see Appendix A) or who is depressed may withdraw to his bedroom to avoid interaction with the nursing staff. On such occasions it is the nurse who initiates and sustains any interaction; she also judges the nature of the interaction. Is it appropriate to converse with the patient or is non-verbal communication sufficient to convey concern and understanding?

It is sometimes difficult to feel you have established contact with a withdrawn person even though interactions have taken place. Furthermore, some people suffering from anxiety states make their need for contact known; others, however, may be left out and their needs missed by staff members. Accordingly some contact should be offered to all patients so that those whose need for interaction is greatest have their need identified and taken into account when planning their care. The appropriate nursing intervention may require contact for as prolonged a period as possible with these patients, and, as stated earlier, this may make an important contribution to their progress. Such planned interventions with patients make considerable emotional demands on the nurse. She tries to help the patient without feeling she has necessarily succeeded, or knowing whether or not her efforts are appreciated. Rejection by the disturbed patient is often very hurtful and it would be easy for the nurse to withdraw, yet what the patient may need is acceptance and perseverance in spite of the rejecting attitude. To withdraw from contact at this point, moreover, may merely serve to reinforce the unhealthy pattern of interaction to which the patient is accustomed.

It is sometimes difficult to tolerate the silent apathy or the unemotional withdrawal of some patients. With such patients, the nurse has to learn the art of being with a person without doing anything at all. Until the person feels psychologically safe with the nurse, quiet companionship may be all that is required.

Non-verbal Interactions

It is not always easy to know whether touching is found to be helpful or not to the patient. When you feel concern, when you want to comfort, you tend to touch people gently or hold their hands. This may be appreciated, for example by the severely depressed or confused person, but others may shrink from touch. Some patients, on the other hand, seek closeness with the nurse. It may then be the nurse who shrinks from such contact and makes the patient feel rejected; this requires careful and thoughtful management.

In conversation or in social activities the physical distance between nurse and patient may be important. Sometimes patients come very much closer to the person to whom they are speaking than is the case among most people. For others the reverse may be true; it is as though they find the closeness of others a threat to their personal space.

Talking with Patients

Most patient–nurse interactions involve talk. It is an essential part of the function of the psychiatric nurse to create opportunities which enable the person to talk as freely as possible. An interested, listening attitude is a necessary beginning but it is not enough. It is also vital to develop special interactive skills (see also below). If the person is to speak freely, the place and the time must be right and the atmosphere conducive to conversation. This is hard to generalize about. Sometimes sitting comfortably in armchairs is right, but sitting down is not always necessary. Some people can talk best while walking up and down the room or the garden. Others talk most freely when in bed in the evening with the night nurse sitting beside them. Some people can talk while having a bath, others may find that the best time for them is to talk over a meal or a cup of tea. Some individuals can only talk openly if they are alone with the nurse, others prefer a group setting—the presence of others can be supportive and can give them courage.

Few people feel able to talk about their feelings as soon

as the approach is made by the nurse though some feel under such pressure to talk that they are constantly in search of a nurse who will listen. Many people, however, need a period of superficial social 'chit-chat' before they can get to any important point they wish to make. Occasionally the person can only speak about important matters at the very end of a period of interaction. When preparations to leave are obvious, the person says: 'Oh, just one more thing . . .' and then proceeds to talk about something which is often highly significant. Because this is known to happen from time to time it may sometimes be appropriate to tell the person the approximate length of time that is available. An example of an opening statement might be: 'We have three-quarters of an hour just now, I was wondering if we could spend the time to talk together, if you wish.' It is also easier to sit with a person in silence if both people know in advance how much time they have together.

Encouraging sounds and nods are often enough to keep the person talking. Sometimes it is necessary to say a little more: 'Go on', 'Yes and then?', 'Tell me more' or 'Would you like to tell me more about this?' Repeating what the person has just said, or perhaps simply rearranging the word order, may help the individual to continue. Acceptance of what the person says as valuable, interesting and important also assists someone to talk freely.

While the person is talking he is sure to watch the nurse's face for signs of approval or disapproval. Neither approval nor disapproval helps. If the patient were to sense moral indignation, disapproval or condemnation, or to feel he has hurt or embarrassed the nurse, he would be likely to stop talking.

If the nurse approves, there is always the danger that sooner or later she will disapprove. For this reason the person may be constantly on the alert to detect whether or not any disapproval might be forthcoming, and may in fact challenge or provoke the nurse to reject him, to disagree or to indicate her disapproval. A non-judgemental acceptance is vital if future interactions and relationships are to be positive experiences for the individual.

Sometimes nurses find quite spontaneously the right words and gestures, the right openings and responses, to make the person feel at ease. More often though, nurses who merely act on intuition and commonsense may find that their responses have reinforced the reaction with which the patient had, before admission, met attempts of help. The nurse's interaction with people should develop into a purposeful activity and planned objectives should be clear in the nurse's mind.

Active Listening Skills

One such objective, as suggested above, may be to provide the person with an *active listener*. Listening closely to what the person says is a very effective means of 'telling' him of your interest and concern, or your wish to understand something of how he feels and of how much you care about his distress (Hardin & Harlaris, 1983). Fully attending to the person's words requires a certain amount of practice by the more inexperienced nurse. Initially concern may focus on trying to think what to say next: she may only be hearing the person speak. But a crucial element of active listening involves learning to keep quiet and not to interrupt. Attentive listening requires the nurse to concentrate on what is being said; she has to be able to paraphrase the gist of what the individual has just been talking about if after a pause he asks: 'What was I saying just now? My mind has gone blank.'

Silences should not be broken simply because the

nurse begins to feel uncomfortable. The patient may be needing to collect his thoughts and to reflect on what he has been disclosing to the nurse—in some cases perhaps it is the first time he has been able to talk of certain matters.

Non-verbal behaviours such as sitting at the same level and leaning towards the person, giving appropriate eye contact—too much may be threatening, too little may indicate the nurse is getting restive—and an interested facial expression, may all reassure the patient that the nurse is attending closely (see also p. 252).

Specific Verbal Responses

There may be occasions when it is appropriate to comment on the patient's non-verbal behaviour. The nurse may say: 'I notice you are biting your upper lip . . . you look tense . . . you seem to have been crying.' 'Would you like to talk?' 'Would it help to tell me?' These might be the kind of remarks which encourage a patient to express his feelings.

It sometimes helps to recognize how painful and distressing things must be for the patient. 'I can see this makes you feel frightened' or 'This has made you feel lonely' may indicate the nurse's sensitivity.

For some patients, the objective is to gain insight; for some, to develop emotional control. It may help the patient if the nurse assists him to look at a problem more closely, to examine it from more points of view, and to express his thoughts about resolving it. If, for example, the person talks about the attitude of his family, it may help to ask him to describe it more fully or to say: 'And how does your sister feel about this?' or to explore a specific incident by asking 'and then what did you say? . . . what did your sister say?'

To help the patient gain emotional control it is sometimes useful to state how the situation is perceived by the nurse, e.g. 'You are angry' or 'You seem to be angry with me', or 'You are angry with me because I did not give in to you' or even 'I have the impression you are doing this to make me angry'. It is almost impossible for the patient to continue behaving in an uncontrolled manner once the difficulty has been recognized and openly stated. (See Chapter 12.)

Talking is not made easier by asking probing questions about the patient's life history or about his emotional difficulties or about his beliefs. Insight is not gained by asking 'Why?' If the patient knew why his behaviour is disturbed, he would not need the nurse's help. He might discover 'Why' if the nurse helps him to explore 'when, where, how, how long, what else, who with'.

Regardless of the setting in which care takes place it is not uncommon for people to ask nurses for advice. Advice is, however, rarely what is needed. Very often the person who asks for advice merely wants someone to confirm that his own decision was the correct one.

It is hardly ever useful to give advice. If it were taken, the person could place the responsibility for his subsequent action on the adviser, whereas the aim is to help the person make his own decision and take responsibility for his own action. Advice given without due consideration of all relevant factors is useless, and conflicting advice undermines an individual's confidence in his carers and increases his difficulties. A nurse who gives advice too readily indicates to the recipient that she considers herself competent to solve a problem which has proved to be a difficulty to him. This attitude may discourage him from further discussion of his problems, which he may feel are not taken seriously enough by the staff.

Of course, a straight refusal to give advice may be resented, as is a refusal to answer direct questions. The nurse can avoid giving advice or answering questions by restating the problem, rephrasing it, trying to get the person to clarify it. A cooperative effort can be made to understand the full implication of any proposed action and to explore the person's feelings about it. In the last resort each individual must feel free to make his own decisions, even his own mistakes.

During prolonged contact with a patient, interactions arise in which the nurse is uncertain how to respond. Inevitably there are moments when her reply is tactless and she becomes aware of having offended the patient. Inevitably her response occasionally has the effect of cutting the patient off. Moments of guilt are bound to occur and there are also periods of frustration when the patient seems to be getting worse rather than better (Pearson, 1990).

Post-interaction Discussion

All learners—and senior nurses too—need the opportunity to discuss with other experienced colleagues the interactions they have with people. Such post-interaction discussion or supervision, when carried out by senior clinical or tutorial staff, is a very valuable learning tool. In preparation for a teaching session, the junior student may sometimes be asked to record immediately after the interaction what the patient said and did, what she said and did in response, and also how the patient reacted. The learner should note how she felt during the interaction and her observations of the patient's feelings.

She may be asked to examine the effect she had on the patient and evaluate the interaction. Such headings may appear on the recording sheet to aid recall. Occasionally, in special circumstances, the interactions may be taped and as with any formal teaching session the person's permission is obtained beforehand.

This practice, known as *process recording*, may be carried out daily over a week or so; each interaction lasts approximately half an hour. Process recordings are useful for helping learners develop their communication skills: the benefits to the patients are perhaps less apparent. However, Nicol and Withington (1981), in a follow-up of a patient–nurse interaction project, comment that 'some (people) said that they found it easier to talk about their problems in group therapy sessions following (one-to-one) discussion with the learner'.

Research by Davis (1986) finds that the 'strain of training' to become a psychiatric nurse can be quite considerable, especially for learners in their first year of the course. One cause of such stress may be from prolonged interactions with patients, particularly those who are most in need of sustained contact. The guidance and support of colleagues must be freely available for the student nurse to enable her to retain her own emotional equilibrium while she is developing her interactive skills.

HUMAN RELATIONSHIPS

After one or two interactions, such as those described above, have taken place, the nurse may feel she is beginning to form a relationship with the patient. The patient, for his part, begins to appreciate the care, concern and interest the nurse shows during the periods of time they spend together. Yuen, (1986) suggests that the nurse–patient relationship is basic to all forms of successful psychiatric nursing care; Barker (1989a) describes it as 'paramount'.

'Good' and 'Bad' Relationships

Nurses sometimes use adjectives like 'good' or 'bad' to qualify the word relationship, when they discuss what happens between the patient and themselves. Such judgements may be invalid, as it is difficult to decribe what kind of relationship is good or bad for the patient. It may be good for the patient to have a negative relationship, for example one of hostility towards a nurse, if this enables him to discuss his feelings, not only about the nurse but about other significant people in his life. It may be bad for the patient to have a positive relationship with a nurse, if such a relationship allows him to remain excessively dependent, or if it prevents exploration of aggressive feelings. More will be said later in this chapter about some of the difficulties surrounding the nurse–patient relationship.

The pattern of relationships into which any person enters changes throughout life. Every contact a person makes contributes something towards the formation of relationships and the quality of every human contact depends to some extent on the relationships which already exist. Without contact with people one cannot learn to relate to them. A child who has very little contact with his mother or father cannot learn to enter into a relationship with them. Only repeated contact with his parents enables the child to develop trust and love, and only repeated contact with the child enables parents to develop the concern and tenderness for their child which are characteristic of good parent–child relationships. When a parent–child relationship has been established, its existence affects every contact the parent and child have with each other. For example, the mother's correction is acceptable to the child or the child's temper is acceptable to the mother because of the relationship which already exists between them. The child allows and expects either his mother or father to bathe him, tuck him up in bed and kiss him, activities which he would resent from a stranger with whom he has no loving relationship.

Relationships between people may be characterized by their emotional content. Loving, caring for, prizing, being concerned, are the positive emotional characteristics; hating, feeling angry, disappointed or frustrated, the negative emotional characteristics of relationships between people.

In the course of life one establishes relationships with people differing in quality, in intensity and in the extent to which they are reciprocated. The relationships between mother and child or between father and child or between siblings may develop into the prototypes of the kind of relationships one enters into later in life. Status determines the rights and obligations of each participant in a relationship. Sibling relationships and friendships are relationships in which the participants' roles and status are similar whereas the parents' status is different from that of their children; the parents' status entitles them to tell them what to do and the children's status obliges them to obey.

Some patients have experienced, in childhood, difficulties in some of their basic relationships. These difficulties may have contributed to disturbed relationships with people in adult life, giving rise to marital problems or difficulty in coping with authority figures such as employers. Experience of life in hospital, and the variety of therapies offered, may enable the patient to learn to deal more effectively with the changing relationships into which he enters on discharge.

Changing Patterns of Nursing Care

When considering the importance given to the establishment of the nurse–patient relationship in present day psychiatric nursing practice, it is difficult to appreciate that the concept is a relatively recent one. At one time, in keeping with the prevailing climate of care based on the management of patients' lives according to rigid routine and rules, the nurse assumed a dominant (parental) and custodial role. For their part, the patients, with little or no opportunity to show initiative, became submissive and apathetic. Fundamental changes in patient care followed the introduction of the therapeutic community approach, and more recently, as discussed in Chapter 4, the nursing process, primary nursing/key worker system and nursing models of care. In psychiatric circles today, practitioners subscribe as we have seen earlier to the view that whenever feasible patients should be partners in actively planning their care. Freedom of expression at ward meetings and group therapy is encouraged, as is one-to-one interaction with a member of the nursing staff and the consequent development of a relationship beneficial to the patient.

Factors Affecting Nurse–Patient Relationships

The Role of Transference

Despite these new patterns of care and an egalitarian milieu, with the use of first names and the absence of uniforms, difficulties in nurse–patient relationships may still occasionally arise. For example, a patient whose earlier problems with an overstrict father or a domineering mother remain unresolved may try to force the nurse into an authoritarian role. In such a situation the nurse could become the target for the patient's negative feelings in place of the parent; i.e. a transference relationship is formed wherein the patient transfers negative feelings for the parent to the nurse.

Awareness and acceptance of the underlying reasons for the patient's antipathy will help the nurse to react positively rather than with a repetition of the authoritarianism the patient has learned to expect from past experiences. Participation in group or individual therapy sessions may allow the patient to achieve an understanding of his or her present behaviour and its relevance to unresolved conflicts.

Patients' Need for Dependency/Friendship

Other patients may expect the nurse to take the part of an all-providing parent figure in a relationship. The patient looks upon the nurse as someone on whom he can depend for the satisfaction of all his needs, while he passively adopts the role of a helpless child. Very occasionally this dependent parent–child relationship is entered into readily by a nurse who is unaware of her own inner need to feel useful and important to someone. Considerable support and guidance from senior colleagues will be necessary to help her recognize and resolve her personal difficulties.

The dependent patient requires encouragement to appreciate the long-term benefits of caring for himself, however reluctant he may be at first to consider this, and however long it may take him to carry out self-care activities. In the equal relationship which gradually develops, the nurse will wish to resist any temptation to make decisions for the patient, to suggest possible solutions when difficulties arise or put forward courses of action which she feels ought to be pursued.

Nurses and adolescent patients sometimes enter into relationships which resemble sibling relationships; if the nurse can fulfil the role of older brother or sister, the patient may benefit by using her as a model on which to pattern his or her own behaviour, or by identifying with her and consequently becoming aware of his or her own positive attributes.

Many patients need friends. Their isolation from people and inability to make and keep friends may be the cause or the result of their present difficulties. The opportunity to find a friend in hospital may be of great therapeutic significance. However, the relationship between the nurse and the patient seldom develops into real friendship. What characterizes friendship is mutual trust and mutual exchange of confidences. Friends make demands on each other and take it for granted that their demands will be met. Friends treat each other as equals, share each other's troubles and difficulties. It is not possible for the nurse to burden the patient with her problems or with her personal affairs, and consequently the relationship becomes one-sided. The choice of meeting places and the duration of interactions is often one-sidely determined to suit the convenience of the nurse not the patient. In conversation between the nurse and the patient the focus is on the need of the patient not the need of the nurse. The relationship between nurse and patient is often of greater importance to the patient than it is to the nurse. To the patient it may seem a unique relationship, but to the nurse the patient is only one of many with whom she relates. Her personal family or friends provide the satisfaction of closer bonds. She does not regard her relationship with the patient as a significant event in her own life and she does not plan that the relationship should continue indefinitely. If the patient regards the relationship with the nurse as a personal, rather than a professional one, he may become disappointed and previous antisocial attitudes may be reinforced.

There are a few occasions when the inexperienced nurse does put herself in the role of friend to the patient, and the actions of a friend come to be expected by the patient. This may be because the patient's suffering is particularly obvious and his appeals for help particularly urgent. The patient may succeed in making the nurse feel sure that she understands him much better than anyone else, and that only she can be relied on to provide the right approach and the right support. This kind of relationship is rarely beneficial to the patient. It leads to increasing demands, and the nurse begins to feel resentful of these demands. The fact that the patient is not responding in a more positive way causes the nurse to feel disappointed and guilty and eventually possibly angry with the patient. Consequently she tends to withdraw her support and the patient feels rejected.

The Concept of 'Over-involvement'

The term 'over-involvement' is sometimes used to describe a relationship in which the nurse's own emotional troubles and unfulfilled needs render her unable to perceive the patient's problems objectively. Kingston (1987) cites an example of a third year student nurse who became over-involved with a depressed patient of about her own age. The student asserted that 'her' patient, with whom she was in the habit of spending long periods of time, and whose situation preoccupied her both on and off duty, was being inadequately treated by the medical team. Subsequently it emerged that the nurse was suffering from depression at the time she was caring for the patient and that she had projected her own need for help onto the patient. In this context, Peplau (1952) points out that it requires 'continual self study by the nurse so that patients are not used to meet our needs', and as stated earlier, a system of personal support for staff has to be available to facilitate the sharing of feelings and difficulties that may arise before a non-therapeutic relationship develops between nurse and patient.

The next part of this chapter considers further the nature of the relationship described earlier as paramount to the successful practice of psychiatric nursing.

Building a Helping Nurse–Patient Relationship

As well as the conversational skills highlighted in the first section of this chapter, some specific nursing skills of value in building a helping relationship will now be outlined.

Ability to Show Empathy, Warmth, Genuineness and Respect

One of the vital components of the helping relationship is the nurse's ability to show *empathy* towards the patient. Empathy may be described as the ability to perceive the meaning of the feelings of another individual and to communicate this understanding to him (Rogers, 1957).

For example, if the nurse responds to the feeling tone behind a depressed person's delusions (see Appendix A) rather than to their content, and feeds back her sensitivity towards his emotional distress, she may be said to be showing empathy. Burnard (1988) when defining empathy asks the nurse to try to enter the patient's 'frame of reference'—to see the world through his or her eyes.

A helping relationship will also be fostered if the nurse shows warmth, genuineness and respect for the patient, and if she accepts uncritically the patient as he is: a unique individual in need of help. The nurse–patient relationship is examined by Barker (1989a) who comments:

> If I 'show' interest in the person I am working with, 'bounce-back' in a creative way some of the things he says for further elaboration, convince him that I have some emotional understanding of his experience, and do not patronise or reject him, I might expect to have a good relationship.

But sometimes it may be difficult for a nurse not to reject a particular patient. If, for example, bitter memories of a parent's frequent outbursts of drunken and violent behaviour are still fresh, it may be hard for her to enter into a helping relationship with someone who had been admitted with an alcohol problem. Open and frank discussions with experienced colleagues are necessary to help this nurse develop an awareness of the influence past experiences play in present perceptions, and of the extent to which an understanding of her own functioning will determine how well she can understand the situation of this patient from *his* point of view. The more the nurse can become involved in trying to understand the patient's world the less she wishes to evaluate it (Rogers, 1957) (see also p. 254).

Ability to Convey Trust

Another of the prerequisites for the development of a helping relationship—and one highly prized by the patient—is the nurse's ability to convince the patient by her actions and responses that she is the kind of person in whom he can place his trust. Trust is conveyed in a variety of ways, some of which include the nurse making sure that:

- information obtained from the patient in confidence is confined to the multidisciplinary team;
- she is consistent with caring and non-judgemental responses;
- she listens attentively to the patient's words;
- when promises are made they are always kept, if at all possible.

Ability to Care

Earlier in this chapter over-involvement and its attendant damaging effects were considered. Such a rare occurrence must be clearly distinguished from the concept of *involvement* and its benefits to the patient. We cannot not become involved: a degree of emotional involvement is a necessary condition for the establishment of a caring relationship between nurse and patient. Without it, the nurse's actions will fail to demonstrate any of the qualities outlined above; indeed the act of caring itself is tantamount to becoming involved. As Anthony (1991) states 'we (patients) need objectivity like a soufflé needs a slab of concrete . . . we *need* people who care'. Also on the theme of caring, Barker (1989b) suggests nurses 'might learn how to care, by learning how to fuse themselves (albeit temporarily) to their patients'; to become so fully absorbed 'in the act of "just listening" or "just talking"' that awareness of 'what makes me and the "patient" different' appears to get lost in the process.

The Concept of Psychological Safety

During the interactions which facilitate the development of the helping relationship the patient may be more able to disclose his true feelings if the nurse can help him feel it is psychologically safe to do so. 'Psychological safety is a difficult concept to define' (Mincardi & Riley, 1988). The following tentative account of its main components also serves to summarize many of the points raised above.

The nurse's use of empathy together with her unfailing support and encouragement can help people feel secure enough to express openly how they feel and to talk freely about their difficulties. Listening attentively, seeking clarification when necessary, not interrupting, accepting uncritically, and respecting their beliefs add to the creation of a 'safe' environment for them. The nurse has also to be able to demonstrate to patients, either verbally or non-verbally, that she cares and is interested in them as people. There ought to be no attempt to advise them on how to solve their problems: rather the nurse provides a psychologically secure setting in which they may begin to seek possible solutions for themselves.

In facilitating patients to disclose their feelings, to work out their own solutions and to be active partners in the planning and implementation of their care, the final stage in the nurse–patient relationship can then be reached. Peplau (1952) describes this stage in the relationship as a 'freeing process'—the time during which both parties in the relationship can withdraw. At this point the patient and the nurse may reflect on the therapeutic developments which it is hoped will have taken place over time. The patient may perhaps now feel better equipped to cope should similar problems arise in the future: the nurse will have gained essential experience to use with subsequent patients.

SUMMARY

This chapter has discussed the nurse's specific role in interacting with people in her care and also the communication skills required to establish a helping relationship with them. Considerable emphasis has been given to the acquisition of such skills; this is deliberate since they are *fundamental* to a positive outcome in the nursing care of the person in need of psychiatric help.

FURTHER READING

Burnard P (1990) *Learning Human Skills*. Oxford: Heinemann.

Crossfield T (1989) How to communicate better. Part 1. *Nursing Standard* 2(22): 39.

Crossfield T (1989) How to communicate better. Part 2. *Nursing Standard* 3(23): 39.

Dexter G & Wash M (1986) *Psychiatric Nursing Skills: A Patient-Centred Approach*. London: Croom Helm.

Egan G (1982) *The Skilled Helper*. New York: Brooks Cole.

Ironbar N & Hooper A (1989) *Self-instruction in Mental Health Nursing*. London: Baillière Tindall.

Koshy K (1989) I only have ears for you. *Nursing Times* 85(30): 26–29.

Kozier B & Erb G (1988) *Concepts and Issues in Nursing Practice*. Wokingham: Addison Wesley.

Reynolds W & Cormack D (eds) (1990) *Psychiatric and Mental Health Nursing*. London: Chapman & Hall.

REFERENCES

Altschul A (1972) *Patient–Nurse Interaction*. Edinburgh: Churchill Livingstone.

Anthony A (1991) Mirror images. *Nursing Times* **87**(2): 35–36.

Barker P (1989a) Rules of engagement. *Nursing Times* **85**(51): 58–60.

Barker P (1989b) Reflections on the philosophy of caring in mental health. *International Journal of Nursing Studies* **26**(2): 131–141.

Burnard P (1988) Empathy: the key to understanding. *Professional Nurse* **3**(10): 388–391.

Davis B (1986) *The Strain of Training: Being a Student Psychiatric Nurse*. In: Brooking J (ed.) *Psychiatric Nursing Research*. Chichester: Wiley.

Dobbin J (1990) First-name terms. *Nursing Times* **86**: 22–34.

Hardin S & Harlaris A (1983) Non-verbal communications of patients and high and low empathy nurses. *Journal of Psychosocial Nursing* **21**(1): 14–20.

Kingston B (1987) *Psychological Approaches in Psychiatric Nursing*. London: Croom Helm.

Mincardi H & Riley M (1988) Providing psychological safety through skilled communication. *Nursing* **3**(27): 990–992.

Nicol E & Withington D (1981) Recorded patient–nurse interactions—an advance in psychiatric nursing. *Nursing Times* **26**(9): 1352.

Pearson M (1990) Small steps to progress. *Nursing Times* **86**(42): 29–30.

Peplau H (1952) *Interpersonal Relationships in Nursing*. New York: Putman.

Rogers C (1957) The necessary and sufficient conditions for personality change. *Journal of Consulting Psychotherapy* **21**: 95–103.

Yuen F (1986) The nurse–client relationship: a mutual learning experience. *Journal of Advanced Nursing* **11**: 529–533.

Chapter 7
Caring for the Person who is Depressed

INTRODUCTION

A distinction needs to be drawn between a true clinical depression and that which most people experience from time to time. Some of the causes of depression will be examined, and consideration given as to how people suffering from depressive illnesses can be cared for in the community, and, in the case of the severely depressed person, in hospital. Their psychological, physical and social needs will all be taken into account throughout the assessment process, leading to a plan of care tailored to each person's individual needs.

Most people have experienced what it feels like to be low in spirits, fed-up, unwilling to get up in the mornings, bored, unable to concentrate for long, unable to tackle the tasks they know they must do. For most people these periods are transitory; they pass and people get on with things. Eventually they recover their usual 'joie de vivre' and are able to enjoy the world around them and the people in it.

People who experience depression or a depressive illness will describe an intensification of all those symptoms, but they do not pass. They persist. People describe a black cloud descending on them; a tight band round their heads. Their normal sleep pattern is disturbed. They lose their appetite and any interest in food and consequently lose weight. They lose all energy. Interest in their appearance and their relationships with family and friends, sense of achievement at work, pleasure in leisure activities, all these cease. In fact, life can become utterly meaningless to them and they begin to long for an escape from this seemingly endless sense of despair and hopelessness.

Causes of Depression

In many cases a reason or cause behind these feelings can be recognized. It is possible to anticipate some of the occasions when people are particularly vulnerable to becoming distressed, times of major change or loss (see Life Events Scale, Appendix D). It is when the body's normal healing abilities fail to adapt to these pressures and stresses that people develop illnesses which may manifest themselves in physical symptoms or in psychological symptoms such as depression.

With other people there appears to be no obvious cause behind the way they are feeling. Everything in their lives appears as normal, with no significant change, but, nevertheless, they feel dreadful. It is sometimes particularly difficult for family and relatives to recognize what is happening as they themselves cannot see an obvious reason to be so miserable and listless. Recent research has found a link between diet and mood (Mackarness, 1976). The depletion of certain chemical neurotransmitters in the brain indicates strong biological factors acting on the brain to cause changes in mood (Henry, 1988; and see Appendix C). Other research has found that people who present with depression have developed a particular way of thinking that distorts reality and their perception of the world around them (Beck, 1976).

Morbidity studies have found that many more women than men present to their GPs complaining of feeling depressed. Reasons suggested for this include the following factors.

- Women tend to describe their feelings more readily and more easily than men.
- A lower status is given to the traditional occupations of women so that they feel undervalued and frustrated when they are bound to the house through motherhood.
- Women become depressed when the normally close relationship with their mothers is no longer available to them, either through moving away from the home environment, or the break-up of family relationships.

There appear to be particular age bands when women present more frequently with depression. The first of these is in early adulthood with the pressures of adjusting to marriage and motherhood without support from one's own family. The second is in middle age when women seem to lose a sense of purpose and usefulness, and the third is in old age. Women have a longer life expectancy than men and find that as they live longer so their physical needs increase; they become more dependent on others; they become more isolated and lonely as their friends and relations either die or move away. The incidence of suicide among the elderly, and in particular among elderly men, is alarmingly high.

Loss in any form, if left unresolved, may lead to people becoming depressed. This is not confined to the loss of a loved person, but can arise from the loss of a job with the possible accompanying loss of income and status that result, loss of a limb through accident or illness, loss of a home or a beloved animal. Murray Parkes (1972) identified four main stages of bereavement: numbness and a state of shock, denial, anger and resolution. Most people are able to work through their grief satisfactorily in time. Sometimes people can become stuck at any one of the stages and need help to accept and come to terms with the loss. The most common stage at which this happens is the anger stage. It can be very difficult and uncomfortable to admit that one feels angry with someone one loves for dying and leaving one behind. People feel guilty, which adds to the anger. It is easier to internalize the hurt and anger on oneself and become depressed and stuck than to allow the expression of the anger and guilt.

People who are abused in childhood frequently grow up with feelings of worthlessness, guilt, shame, inadequacy, with low self-esteem and low self-worth. They have difficulty in sustaining lasting relationships and frequently find themselves choosing the same type of person that abused them in the past. They appear to perpetuate the pattern of unsatisfactory relationships which in turn reinforces their feelings of helplessness and hopelessness (Jehu, 1988).

The Needs of the Depressed Person

Psychological Needs

Feelings, thoughts, reactions, relationships, which can be so puzzling and illogical at times, are complex areas of life's experience. People find it immensely difficult to face up to feelings and thoughts and to discuss them openly with those to whom they should be addressed. Time and opportunity must be offered to them to explore their feelings and thoughts in a safe and confidential setting, whether at home, in a clinic or in hospital. Relationships often break down because there is a failure to communicate between people, a failure to listen to and consider what is being said, a fear of what the reaction may be, a fear of being misunderstood or ridiculed. Depressed people lose confidence in themselves and in their ability to deal with things which normally would not be a problem. They need help and encouragement to regain their normal confidence, or to develop a new-found confidence with which to deal with life.

Physical Needs

Whatever the cause may be, the suffering of people with depression is intense. They will need much patience and loving understanding from those around them. For a while they may need others to take on their daily responsibilities. They may need help with all or some of the things we take for granted, such as washing and dressing themselves, eating a regular diet, taking exercise. One of the common accompaniments of depression is constipation, caused by a combination of poor nutrition and lack of exercise, which can lead to a pre-occupation with physical symptoms or 'psychosomatic' symptoms. Their sleep pattern may be disturbed. If their depression is a reaction to a life event they may have difficulty getting off to sleep and find themselves thinking too much of their worries and troubles. If their depression is of the biological kind they may find themselves waking early in the morning when the intensity of their misery is at its worst. They may both benefit for a short time in taking prescribed medication to enable them to return to a regular sleep pattern. However, one of the dangers which nurses have to avoid is that of encouraging unnecessary dependence on medication such as sleeping tablets. Society has become very aware of the risk of addiction resulting from the abuse of some of the drugs that used to be prescribed on a long-term basis, for example some of the hypnotics and anxiolytics, which have compounded some people's difficulties.

Sociological Needs

Research has found that people who are on low incomes or who are unemployed, who live in sub-standard housing in inner-city deprived areas, who come from ethnic minority groups and who no longer have access to supportive, extended families are more likely to suffer from mental illness (Brown & Harris, 1978). They are less likely to have the inner resources to cope with the stresses that come with major life events, such as illness, loss, whether of job, home, or a loved person. When someone presents with depression it will be necessary to consider all the following areas of their life:

- housing situation
- employment
- finances
- support network
- relationships in the home
- whether the person lives alone
- whether the person or partner has experienced any major life event recently such as: bereavement, loss of job, illness

NURSING THE DEPRESSED PERSON IN THE COMMUNITY

This section considers what is required of the nurse to care for people with depression in the community.

How does a nurse become aware of the depressed person in the community? Any member of a primary health care team may refer a person to the Community Mental Health Team requesting a mental health assessment. Let us assume that it is agreed that the community psychiatric nurse (CPN) should visit the referred client at home. The CPN may choose to collect as much information as possible from the GP and referrer before making the visit. On the other hand, the CPN may prefer to visit with a clear and unbiased mind, so as to observe and discuss with the client what the problems and difficulties really are. So often one finds that people present with one list of problems to their GP but on investigation and careful questioning all sorts of other problems surface. By visiting clients in their own home and on their own territory, where they feel more relaxed and confident enough to bring up underlying areas of concern, the CPN will be able to make a fuller assessment. If at all possible the CPN will want to meet other members of the family to try to obtain as complete a picture as possible of the situation and the circumstances which may be contributing to the depression. There may be financial worries which the husband and wife feel unable to discuss together; there may be problems with one or more of the children; there may be trouble with unsatisfactory housing conditions; difficulties at work that require courage and determination to tackle; a breakdown in their ability to talk honestly together, dissatisfaction in their sexual relationships, usually resulting from a lack of understanding and patience with one another which leads to more unhappiness. There could be any number of contributory factors which the CPN may be able to unravel, and, together with the client, look at ways of overcoming the difficulties.

With the knowledge and skill that comes with training

and experience the CPN will be able to assess whether the person's mental state is such that a discussion with the GP and a suggestion of medication is enough or whether the client should be seen by a psychiatrist. Anti-depressant medication can be an essential part of treatment of the depressed person in the community, and, if successful, can often prevent a worsening of symptoms and avoid the need to go into hospital. It can produce uncomfortable side-effects, which, if not fully explained, can lead to people stopping medication too soon with a return of the symptoms of the depression. By agreeing to visit on a regular basis the CPN can enter into a partnership with the person and together explore what is causing the depression and work out strategies to over-come the identified problems. The CPN will monitor the progress and recovery of the person and answer any questions and allay any anxiety. At the same time the CPN may become involved in:

- counselling;
- offering therapy, if properly trained and supervised. This could be using a behavioural, cognitive or psychodynamic approach;
- offering to work with the family;
- enabling other appropriate agencies to help overcome practical problems, e.g.:
  - social services,
  - housing departments,
  - employers;
- encouraging the client to take on new interests and to meet other people.

All these interactions are directed to enabling people to cope with the difficulties that arise in their lives so that they may feel more fulfilled, less isolated and more con-fident in themselves.

The Risk of Suicide

There will be times when people do not respond to medication in the community, when their carers are no longer able to guarantee their safety, and when the future looks so bleak and hopeless to them that they speak of wanting to commit suicide. They may have become so despairing that the only solution to them is to commit suicide. Without any obvious warning they make an attempt. In these situations there is usually no alternative but to admit them to hospital, wherever possible with their agreement and consent. If they are still determined to kill themselves it may become necessary to use a section of the Mental Health Act to remove them to a place of safety until they are sufficiently recovered and no longer actively seeking to die. (The care these people will require on admission to hospital is examined later in this chapter.) Any talk of wanting to die must be taken very seriously by all mental health workers, especially when people with a known history of depression speak in these terms. With the benefit of hindsight, relatives and carers have said that they could have recognised signs that indicated an intention of being about to commit suicide.

Community psychiatric nurses, along with all mental health workers, need to be skilled in assessing suicide risk. They must know what questions to ask and how to ask them. They must be able to recognize the signs that indicate whether a depressed person is contemplating ending his life. By careful questioning the CPN can discover the means by which people are planning to kill themselves. Those who describe the more violent means, such as shooting themselves, hanging, drowning, throwing themselves in front of trains and motor vehicles, tend to be those at greatest risk of succeeding.

People living in rural areas where the presence and use of shotguns are a normal and accepted way of life can be tempted to use them against themselves in their despair. Farmers are amongst the third highest category of people who commit suicide. As the availability of firearms becomes so much more widespread within the population as a whole, the CPN will need to make very careful and thorough arrangements with members of the family or friends that firearms are kept locked away or removed entirely from the home until the person is feeling well again. When people express suicidal thoughts, ideas or intentions the CPN has to decide whether it is safe for each individual to remain at home, or whether it is safer and better for that individual to go into hospital. The CPN will need to consult with the GP and with the psychiatrists in the team if there is any cause for doubt or uncertainty as to each person's safety. This is where it is so important to work with families and friends who can arrange to spend time with the depressed person, and to liaise closely with both the GP and the specialist mental health team. It may be necessary for the CPN to visit very frequently for a period until the person begins to feel better.

However, experience has shown that when people are deeply depressed and wish to kill themselves they often lack the energy and motivation, but as their mood lifts and they feel less inertia, they find the will to act on their ideas. This can be an extremely dangerous time and all nurses need to be alert to the possibility that people recovering from a severe depression may carry out the desire to kill themselves.

Some people do not really want to die but are unable to see a sensible way of solving their difficulties. They feel unable to say outright what their problem really is. They make suicidal gestures. They take an overdose of tablets.

They cut their wrists. They become drunk and behave in an irresponsible manner. This type of behaviour is often described as being a 'cry for help', an attempt to attract attention to the fact that they are in distress, unable to cope, or are in need of help of some kind. It is very tempting when working in a busy and hard-pressed Accident and Emergency Department to be dismissive and irritated with these people, especially when the same people return time after time. But it is these very people who may be most damaged by their early experiences. They have learned unsatisfactory ways of dealing with stress and require the greatest patience and understanding to help them in their distress. They need the opportunity to learn more satisfactory ways of coping with situations and circumstances that they find difficult. They need to learn self-esteem and self-worth; they need to feel confident and competent to control their own lives and be responsible for themselves. In order to achieve this they need to understand what has contributed to the unsatisfactory patterns of behaviour they have adopted. This may involve reliving some of the very painful and frightening feelings that accompanied those early experiences. Some people will find it too traumatic to explore those feelings and will continue to react in their unhappy way. Those people who do wish to overcome their difficulties will require great sensitivity from the nurse who is working with them. They must feel trust and confidence that the nurse will not be judgemental, but will accept them and want to work with them.

Likewise, nurses need help to recognize that the different expressions of suicidal intent may represent a continuum as to the risk to life, on the one hand a 'cry for help' at times of distress and on the other a very real and determined desire to end one's life. Many people will experience elements along the continuum, at different levels of intensity at different times, depending on their own individual circumstances. Nurses need to learn that all people who express a wish to end their lives need to be looked after and cared for in such a way as to enable them to regain a sense of self-worth and a purpose in living.

CARE STUDY 1

Mrs Elizabeth K.

Age: 54 years.

Married for 28 years to Richard, an electrical engineer.

Three children: Paul aged 26 years, Andrew aged 24 years and Jennie aged 21 years.

Father died six years ago of a heart attack aged 75 years.

Mother, 79 years old, is less able to cope in the family home, and has decided to sell the house and move into a warden controlled bungalow in the same town as Mrs K, twenty minutes walk away from her home which often necessitates driving.

Elder brother lives far away in the north of England, with whom she has sporadic contact.

Younger brother lives an hour's drive away.

Younger sister lives in London and has a very busy, successful career.

Mrs K herself used to be a very well-respected and competent teacher, both before her marriage and until two years ago when she first developed a depressive illness. She lost confidence in herself and in her ability to control a classroom of students. She began to feel near to tears most of the time, and gradually became easily reduced to tears. She felt worse in the evenings and found it difficult to get off to sleep so that she began to dread the nights; her thoughts would go round and round as she thought of all the things she should have done and which she used to accomplish so easily and efficiently before she became depressed. She has lost her appetite, and only picks at her food. She can still manage to cook a simple meal for her family. As she has been feeling unwell for two years now, in spite of antidepressant medication from her GP, she has agreed to see the community psychiatric nurse who liaises with the practice. Mrs K in the past adamantly refused to see anyone from the specialist mental health service because she had felt so strongly that she should be able to overcome her thoughts and feelings herself. Now she was feeling so hopeless of ever being better that she had begun to have thoughts of harming herself.

The GP had written a letter, referring Mrs K to the CPN. The CPN had contacted Mrs K and they had arranged for the CPN to visit her at home.

Initial Assessment Visit

After introductions and a brief general discussion the CPN explained why she was there and that she hoped they would be able to work together to enable Mrs K to feel better and return to enjoying life again. In order to achieve this the CPN would need to establish with Mrs K just what were her problems, what she had done about them in the past and what she felt able to do about them now. In the course of the session it became apparent that Mrs K had been very close to her father. When he died, her mother had been so distressed that for a while Mrs K had had to spend much time helping and supporting her.

Soon after her mother was able to manage again, her eldest son had broken a leg in a car accident, just as he was about to sit his finals at University and her daughter was in a very anxious state as she was due to sit her GCSE exams. Mrs K had rallied to help them both through this difficult time for them, thus postponing any time to mourn her father's death.

Now that her mother had decided to sell the family home this had brought back the sense of loss for her father and reinforced the knowledge that her mother was becoming older and frailer and would die sooner or later, leaving Mrs K, in her own mind, alone and unsupported. She felt that all the happy memories and the feelings of security that the house had given her over the years would be lost.

She felt overwhelmed at times that she would never be able to cope with looking after her mother when she came to live in the town. Her three children were all grown up, and although her daughter was still living at home she was talking of moving out to share a flat with a couple of friends. There seemed to be a paradox: on the one hand she felt she was no longer any use to her family, and on the other she felt she could not cope with the extra demands that her mother might make on her.

The symptoms experienced by Mrs K were as follows:

- sadness, with a sense of loss, feelings of being close to tears most of the time and being easily reduced to tears;
- feelings of guilt and worthlessness;
- lack of energy, feeling listless and apathetic;
- no interest in doing anything;
- very little concentration;
- preoccupation with thoughts of her worthlessness;
- loss of interest in food with loss of appetite and some weight loss;
- inability to go to sleep with ruminative thoughts of all the things she should have done during the day;
- mood becoming steadly worse as the day proceeds;
- all these things combining to cause a growing sense of hopelessness with more thoughts of wanting to end her life.

The CPN felt considerably concerned about the picture presented by Mrs K and asked her whether she felt she should go into hospital for a while to be cared for until she felt more hopeful about her life. Mrs K repeated what she had said to her GP, that she really did not want to go into hospital. The CPN then questioned her very closely about her suicidal thoughts, and whether she had given any thought to just how she might end her life. At this stage Mrs K had only thought in general terms about wanting to be dead. She had not planned what she might do. The CPN then discussed with Mrs K what they could do together, but stressed that she would need to speak with Mrs K's husband and daughter so that they could all help together and be aware of the intensity of Mrs K's distress. They then listed all the problem areas as felt by Mrs K and put them into a priority order.

Psychological and social needs:

1 To give expression to her feelings of loss and bereavement
   (a) father;
   (b) family home;
   (c) children grown up and leaving home.
2 To overcome feelings of worthlessness, loss of confidence (doubts that she will ever be able to return to full-time teaching).
3 To experience a sense of accomplishment (Mrs K lacks energy and the ability and interest to carry out everyday tasks; everything seems to be a huge effort and she is left with feelings of exhaustion).

Physical needs:

1 To establish a more normal sleep pattern.
2 To avoid further weight loss from a lack of interest in food.

Having agreed what the main areas of need were, the CPN and Mrs K looked at the various alternatives available to meet them.

- As the CPN had attended two courses on bereavement counselling run by the local branch of CRUSE Mrs K was offered either to be referred to CRUSE or to work with the CPN.
- The CPN also described some of the principles underlying the cognitive behaviour therapy approach to coping with depression. At first Mrs K expressed doubts about ever feeling any better, but with gentle patience and the CPN giving clear, simple illustrations of how the approach can work Mrs K agreed to try (see Chapter 13).
- They then established the homework that Mrs K would attempt before the next appointment, having agreed that for the first two weeks the CPN would visit twice a week. Then Mrs K would begin to attend the Mental Health Centre where the CPN was based, partly to help overcome some of Mrs K's prejudice towards all things psychiatric and partly to give her a motive for going out.
- The CPN suggested that Mrs K should see her GP again and try a short course of sleeping tablets to help her to return to a more normal sleeping pattern but at the same time suggested that she learn some relaxation and thought distraction techniques to break the habit of ruminating over the day's activities.
- Although Mrs K's appetite was poor, the CPN suggested that she should not expect to eat a normal quantity at each meal but to give herself small helpings and gradually increase them as she began to feel better.
- The CPN then went over once again what they had agreed, giving a broad outline of the expectations of progress without putting unrealistic pressure on Mrs K.
- They arranged that both Mr K and the daughter would be

present at the next appointment so that the CPN could explain the treatment programme to them and give them all a written care plan to which they could refer and which they could use to evaluate progress.

- They established that Mrs K would start by keeping a chart of how she spent her week, giving a rating of the amount of pleasure and feeling of achievement she experienced for each activity.
- At the next meeting they would begin to look in more detail at the 'negative automatic thoughts' that popped into her head as she went about the day's activities. They would explore these in the course of treatment and Mrs K would learn ways of challenging them that would help her to think more realistically about herself and her future.

The CPN and Mrs K continued to work together for a period of 18 weeks, at the end of which Mrs K had worked through most of her feelings of loss and had learned to accept the changes in her life and to make positive plans for her mothers's move, engaging the help and support of the other members of her family. She had returned to teaching and felt much more confident in her abilities to control the students (she had never had any problem with this before her illness and had learned to accept that it was a consequence of her illness that she felt incompetent). As she had begun to challenge her negative automatic thoughts and to tackle tasks one at a time, so her feelings of worthlessness had diminished and she had soon begun to feel less hopeless about her future. At the end of the treatment programme they agreed that the CPN would contact Mrs K by phone after three months to hear how she was progressing. If in between times Mrs K wished to speak with the CPN she was very welcome to phone at any time. In fact, there had been no need and at the three-month follow-up Mrs K had maintained her improvement. She had helped her mother to move house even though their old home remained unsold. Her daughter had gone ahead with her plans to move into a flat with friends and Mrs K was able to see that as a positive move to greater independence. She and her husband were planning a holiday abroad together, something they had never managed before. As she was over 55 years she was beginning to think of retiring from teaching and taking up some adult education classes at the local community college instead. She was able to see a fairly rosy future for herself, over which she had much more control and choice, and she was feeling a great deal happier with herself and her situation.

CARE STUDY 2

Mrs Margaret P.
Age: 26 years.
Married for five years to John, a long distance lorry driver.
Two children: Gemma aged 2½, Tom aged 15 months.
Parents live in Streatham, London.
Parents-in-law live in Devon.
Margaret has one younger sister still living at home.
Husband, John, comes from a large family but all live in the West Country or overseas.
Mr and Mrs P moved to their present home in the Midlands nine months ago as John's firm is based there.

Margaret has found it very difficult to settle into her new surroundings. With two very young children and a new home to organize she has not been able to get out much to meet other young mothers. Her husband is away much of the week driving to the continent and is tired on his return home. He appears reluctant to help her very much with the children but expects her to pay attention to him and his own need of her.

She herself feels tired, has been alone with the children all week and expects him to amuse and entertain her, or at least to show an interest in what she has been doing all week and to understand some of her frustrations in having to cope with running the house and looking after the children virtually single-handed. She has become irritable towards him, tearful, miserable. She has spoken to her health visitor and to her GP. Both feel that referral to the commuty psychiatric nurse is appropriate.

The CPN Visits to Carry out an Initial Assessment

The two young children are present throughout the interview and constantly demand attention from their mother as she tries to explain her feelings and situation to the CPN. She is frequently in tears and appears upset to be so distressed in front of her children. There is a pile of washing waiting to be ironed on a chair, toys scattered about the floor, a half-finished baby's bottle on the table. She describes how constantly tired she feels, how the housework gets her down and although she knows she should keep the house clean for the children and that she should tidy away the toys which could be a hazard to them, she cannot find the energy to attend to these things. She does make sure that the children are fed, and she tries to take them out for a walk most days. She feels very alone, as she has been unable to make friends yet with any of her neighbours or with any other groups of young mothers. She does phone her mother regularly, but her husband has complained at the cost of their telephone bill. She has been unable to tell him just how miserable she really feels as he has said that she must snap out of being so apathetic.

The CPN tries to ascertain from Margaret what she believes her main problems to be and together they make a list.

- Loneliness with no-one to talk to apart from the children.
- Deteriorating relationship with her husband due in part to her inability to communicate her feelings to him.
- Lack of energy, constant feelings of tiredness, inability to keep on top of the housework.
- Missing contact with any of her family, and not wanting them to know how she is not coping, especially as they did not altogether approve of her marriage to John.

They then begin to explore what Margaret feels she would like to do about each of these problems; in other words they consider the various options open to Margaret.

Option 1: As she is unaware of what is available in the town, the CPN is able to inform her of such groups as a mother and toddler group that some of the local mothers had started and run as a self-help group. The health visitor drops in on a regular basis to give them support and information in case any of them have a particular problem with the children. The CPN and social worker run a group for people who are experiencing depression and anxiety. They are able to provide a crèche facility for those with young children, where the children are looked after by a child-minder for the duration of the group. It always finishes with a cup of tea or coffee before everyone disperses, so giving them an opporunity to gain confidence in a social setting.
Agreed action: For Margaret to join the support group run by the CPN and social worker in order to gain a little confidence and feel better in herself before considering joining the mother and toddler group, but to begin negotiations and meet with the leader of the group.

Option 2: The question of her deteriorating relationship with her husband causes her much anxiety. The CPN suggests that she must start to be more honest with him and let him know how she is feeling. The CPN offers to meet with them both to try to explore what they can do together to improve the relationship.

Agreed action: That Margaret would have a proper talk with her husband and see what his reaction was to meeting with the CPN.

Option 3: As Margaret feels she is not coping with the day-to-day running of the house the CPN suggests that she looks at exactly what she does do each day and keeps a diary for a week. She can try making a list of all the things that she would like to do each day, being realistic in what she should expect to achieve in a day. She should include in her day's list some things that are not chores but things that could be enjoyable interludes or rewards for achieving the chores. There could be enormous pleasure and satisfaction in crossing off each task as it is accomplished.

Agreed action: To keep a diary for a week until their next appointment.

Option 4: As she is missing her family so much, the CPN discusses with Margaret whether there is any possibility of her going to stay for a short period when her husband is on one of his longer trips abroad. Margaret thinks that there would be problems in organizing this at present but it is something she would love to do.

Agreed action: To keep this in mind for when she feels better able to cope with organizing it.

Option 5: The CPN will visit every week for a month and then review how Margaret is feeling, with a view to reducing visits to every fortnight, depending on progress.

This plan was implemented. Within a month Margaret felt able to join the mother and toddler group where she soon made friends with the other mothers. The two children flourished among the other youngsters and became more manageable as Margaret gained confidence in herself. She regained her ability to run and organize her home, and was much less distressed if she did not achieve every thing that she had set herself to do. It was a little more difficult to engage her husband in regular sessions as his work took him away so much, but he appeared genuinely surprised at the depth of Margaret's feelings. He explained that as he came from a large family and his mother had always seemed to cope, so he thought Margaret could and should cope. He admitted that perhaps he had been thoughtless and insensitive. Together they agreed to try to make more time for each other. He would spend more time with the children when he was at home, thus giving her more of a break, and they would begin to plan how to set aside time to do things as a family group.

In this care study the CPN did not adopt quite such a structured approach as in the first, but still tried to be systematic in identifying the problems and in considering the options with which the client was prepared to work. Evaluation took place on every visit through feedback on progress between visits and in monitoring Margaret's mental state, mood, appearance, state of the house, interaction with the children and so forth.

CARING FOR THE SEVERELY DEPRESSED PERSON IN HOSPITAL

The psychological needs of the depressed person will be discussed first followed by his physical and social needs. As has already been pointed out, however, it is somewhat arbitrary to separate a person's needs into three groups since considerable overlap often occurs. It is also essential that if the severely depressed person's physical health has been seriously neglected prior to admission and if he is at risk of harming himself, physical needs will then be a priority. The crucial need for a safe environment for the person who is actively suicidal will be included when this aspect of care is examined later.

Identification of Needs and Nursing Interventions

Psychological Needs

To Feel a Sense of Worth as a Person

The poor sense of worth experienced by deeply depressed people is symptomatic of their feelings of inadequacy and helplessness, and of seeing themselves as a burden to family and friends. Trying to understand how they feel, empathizing with them, is an important first step towards meeting their psychological needs. This can be very difficult if the person is withdrawn, uncommunicative and lacks any interest in what is going on in the unit. On meeting someone who is depressed for the first time, the student nurse may be forgiven for thinking it would perhaps be better if he were to be left alone with his morbid thoughts, since he may scarcely, if at all, acknowledge her presence. Yet those who have recovered from severe depression have spoken of how comforting it was simply to have the physical presence of another human being sitting with them when in despair: Peplau (1952) calls this the 'nearness of the nurse'. On such occasions conversation might seem obtrusive and inappropriate and non-verbal communication such as the nurse placing her arm gently round the person's shoulders can be equally effective in conveying concern. Such gestures may also help to raise the person's self-esteem, if only fleetingly.

Burton (1991), herself a nurse who became depressed, confirms the validity of these interventions:

> 'I needed those who understood enough to reach out to me, be with me. At times a sympathetic presence was enough, at others I needed the comfort of physical contact. A light touch might be sufficient, although there were times when a nurse sat close by me and put her arm around me. A hug will give simple comfort—when words are inadequate that is what you need.'

Sometimes depressed people experience a slight uplift in mood in the evening. In view of this the nurse can use this time of day to talk with the person about his interests and hobbies, having obtained information about them earlier from relatives. The person may possibly feel slightly less negative about himself if he knows that the nurse is concerned enough to take the trouble to find out such personal details of special importance to him.

Additionally nurses are sometimes able to bolster confidence a little and dispel some of the depressed person's thoughts of uselessness and inadequacy by encouraging him to help with ward tasks and by working alongside him giving appropriate praise and thanks afterwards. But it is very important that the nurse takes care to tailor such tasks to suit the person's ability to concentrate. Concentration can be very poor in severe depression and failure could further confirm the depressed person's poor sense of worth; it may also be possible for failure to reinforce a current delusion (a fixed false belief—see below) that, say, his brain is gradually rotting away if unable to play a fairly simple card game. On the other hand a sense of achievement can be gained from as basic a task as making a cup of coffee for a visiting relative, with the nurse's encouragement.

Often depressed people can find it difficult to summon up any energy or enthusiasm to care for their appearance and need a lot of gentle prompting by the nurse. Relatives can be helped to feel less inadequate and more involved in care if invited to bring to the ward the depressed person's favourite toiletries or clothing. If the nurse can then gently persuade the person to use them, the improvement in appearance can prompt favourable comments from others; such positive feedback may help further nurture a more positive self-image. Indecision is often a feature of depression, but with the nurse's support people who are depressed can be allowed to make as many decisions as possible, however trivial, about their care. Again this may help boost self-esteem and lessen feelings of inadequacy.

To Have Delusions Responded to Therapeutically

A delusion may be defined briefly as a fixed false belief, held with unshakeable conviction, and one which cannot be changed by logical argument. Delusions, when present in severe depression, usually reflect the person's prevailing mood of unremitting gloom and self-deprecation.

When someone talks about a delusion of wickedness, for example, it is not appropriate for the nursing staff to behave as though he has not spoken and to respond with a change of subject; nor is it therapeutic to reinforce the delusion in any way or to argue with the content. Rather it is preferable to respond to the feeling tone behind the words and acknowledge empathetically the obvious distress this false belief is causing the speaker: the nurse may add that though she cannot share the delusional idea, she does nevertheless appreciate his need to believe it is true. An explanation from the nurse linking the depressed person's delusion to his severely depressed mood—adding that it is hoped it will become gradually less troublesome and distressing as his state of mind improves—may also be helpful.

As soon as appropriate the nurse may then invite the depressed person to join in some simple diversional activity; in effect attempting to focus his thoughts on reality rather than leaving him to continue to dwell on his delusional thoughts.

To Unlearn Thinking Exclusively Pessimistic Thoughts

A severely depressed person experiences pessimistic thoughts and can become morbidly preoccupied with them to the exclusion of optimistic ones. He has learned that the future holds nothing but terrible suffering. Thus directly a depressed person feels able to venture spontaneously from his usual seat—the chair in the corner of the room isolated from others—he is encouraged to start unlearning this negative way of thinking. For example, the person's primary nurse, knowing of his fondness for music, makes a point of discussing with him the possibility of his attending the twice-weekly musical appreciation sessions, in the hope of getting him to concede that this might be something to look forward to with a degree of pleasure.

Gradually more time is spent each evening discussing together the events of the day. With prompting from the nurse, the depressed person is encouraged to highlight the positive happenings in the hope of beginning a process of what has been called 'optimistic self-grooming' (Gray, 1983).

Physical Needs

To be Cared for in a Safe Environment

The feelings of hopelessness, misery and despair which engulf those who suffer deep depression necessitate their being closely supervised until their mood improves. Nursing staff must make regular checks on their whereabouts throughout the day and night (see p. 59). As a first step towards ensuring the person's safety two nursing team members should look through the person's belongings most carefully on admission. This is also necessary to provide a record of valuables etc. Potentially harmful articles and supplies of medication, which may be brought by those who are depressed, should all be taken into safe keeping. This procedure is carried out after a full and sensitive explanation is given of the reasons why it is necessary, and with the newly-admitted person's permission and cooperation if possible.

For many people it can be quite upsetting to have to allow strangers access to personal belongings; on the other hand it may be reassuring to know that someone cares sufficiently to take such stringent precautions to ensure their well-being while they feel so wretched.

Nurses sometimes find this task embarrassing and for this reason might be tempted to hurry over it. Half-hearted attempts to look at belongings do nothing to alleviate distress or inspire confidence. If the nurses fail to discover harmful objects the person may well feel less safe when with them and consequently more anxious.

Other precautionary measures include the presence of a nurse when the deeply depressed person is bathing and also when spending time in the kitchen for any reason.

Close attention is paid when all medication is administered to make sure drugs are swallowed and not removed from the mouth later, hoarded, then taken in overdose. Liquid preparations can be useful if there is any doubt at all about compliance. Altschul (1985) confirms the therapeutic value of adhering to these caring interventions: 'I felt safe in a place where the nurses knew what I was doing, where people seemed to care about my safety and where someone could always be found for a quiet chat or just sitting beside.'

Unfailing concern by the nursing team for a depressed person's welfare may also be of some help in partially counteracting feelings of unworthiness and for raising self-esteem—an important psychological need discussed earlier. Paradoxically, extra vigilance is required when depressed people begin to emerge slowly from the depths of despair. The inactivity and apathy which hitherto characterized their behaviour gives way to the first stirring of energy which may provide the impetus to harm themselves. This 'initial recovery' coincides with the first two or three treatments of electroconvulsive therapy (ECT) (see p.268) or the first week or so of the administration of antidepressant drugs. But it is essential the nurse recognizes that in both instances *any appreciable improvement in mood lags behind this increase in motor behaviour*.

Drug therapy may present further safety hazards for the elderly person who is depressed. Postural hypotension, and difficulty in initiating micturition in men, are both among the unwanted effects of some antidepressants; the night nurse has to be especially aware of the danger of falls when an elderly man gets up to the toilet in the early hours.

Caring for the person who is actively suicidal. Fortunately severely depressed people usually improve (see care study below), though without active treatment this may take a long time. With skilled nursing care, and often antidepressant therapy—and sometimes ECT—recovery takes place more quickly. But a few severely depressed people may not improve, rather their depression deepens to the point of becoming actively suicidal. The needs of this person do not differ substantially from those of the severely depressed person except for the more stringent measures to be taken to ensure a safe environment known as *maximum* (or *constant*) *observation*. This requires a member of the nursing team to remain with the person round-the-clock and during this time the patient should never be out of sight or out of reach of the nurse.

It is impossible to keep a patient under constant observation without his knowing that this is being done. The nurse should therefore meet the patient's questions frankly, and either herself explain the procedure to him or make sure that his doctor has done this. The patient may still ask the reason for the surveillance, but is then merely expecting the nurse to confirm reasons well known to him. With a little tact the nurse can usually manage to obtain from him the explanation of why he is being observed and so avoid the embarrassment of pretending not to know.

Constant observation is an extremely arduous duty which should be shared. For part of the day it may be possible to keep the patient occupied; games of chess, card games, reading aloud, may make his and the nurse's life easier. It is more difficult if the patient, being deeply depressed, does not wish to speak or be spoken to. There may be long periods of silence and complete inactively on the patient's part, during which the nurse must keep herself occupied, without ever relaxing vigilance. She must not become so absorbed in any work that she will not notice the patient's every movement, yet she cannot just sit and stare at him. The patient has little to do other than watch the staff, and any carelessness or negligence on the part of the nurse is noticed and use may be made of this knowledge at some later date.

Constant observation is specially difficult if the patient shows resentment at the nurse's presence and reacts by totally ignoring or verbally abusing her. It is helpful if the nurse can appreciate the frustrations felt by the patient and understand that his reactions are not directed to her personally but to the world at large. The patient is more likely to react negatively if he feels the nurse is regarding the time spent with him as her spell of 'guard duty'.

On the other hand, being with the patient in this way can provide the nurse with an excellent opportunity to convey her genuine concern and interest in his welfare, such as actively listening if he wishes to talk. Evenings are often the time of day when the patient may feel best able to express his feelings, coinciding as it sometimes does with a slight improvement in mood. Salmons (1984) in a study of suicidal behaviour suggests that the lack of deaths occurring in the period from 6 p.m. till midnight might be a possible reflection of this phenomenon in depression.

When a patient in the ward makes a suicidal attempt, or when a suicide has occurred, repercussions may be evident among patients and staff. Nurses may feel guilty at what they perceive to be a failure in their task of pre-serving life. They feel despondent and distressed, and however earnestly they may try to spare the other patients' feelings, their own emotions inevitably affect ward atmosphere.

There are usually a few patients who share in the self-reproach and guilt feelings of the nursing staff and who believe they might have been able to prevent the tragedy had they been more observant or more ready to confide in the staff that they knew of the patient's suicidal intentions.

Open discussion of the incident afterwards is invaluable. Smyth and Craddock (1989) cite several advantages to be gained from this practice, the first and most important being to help the responsible team to learn lessons from the incident for the benefit of future patients. If conducted sensitively such discussions may relieve, rather than increase, the nurses' and doctors' anxieties.

The incident is also freely discussed at the daily meeting to give patients the opportunity to ventilate their feelings and to put forward constructive and practical ideas on how future attempts might be prevented.

To Maintain a Reasonable Level of Mobility

Unless given a lot of psychological support and encouragement from the nurse, the person who is severely depressed may seldom stir from the chair he occupies in an isolated corner of the day room. He feels lethargic and finds any activity he has to carry out, for example getting up in the morning, a major effort. Persuading the patient to assist with simple ward chores will help meet mobility needs as well as helping his psychological need to feel less inadequate. Winokur (1981) suggests that, as with anxiety and tension states, any form of physical exercise has a beneficial effect on a person's low mood. Short walks out of doors accompanied by a nurse may also help stimulate the depressed person's poor appetite a little, as well as creating a certain degree of well-being, if only temporarily.

*To Take an Adequate Diet and Re-establish Normal
Elimination Patterns*

Many deeply depressed people are too apathetic or morbidly preoccupied to want to eat. They simply do not
want to be bothered, have no desire for food.

Delusions of poverty and unworthiness may also
influence this reluctance to eat. The person may believe
he does not have the money for the food and cannot eat
what he cannot pay for, or else he does not deserve it,
that others are starving; the food should be given to
them. These idea expressed or kept secret, effectively
deter the severely depressed person from eating. The
delusion that he has 'no inside' that his 'bowels are
blocked', may also lead to refusal of food. Or he may feel
that life is no longer worth living and hope to starve
himself to death. The person's unwillingness to eat may
also be due to the somatic (also known as vegetative)
symptoms which accompany major depressive disorders. For example, there is a decrease in the normal
secretion of gastric juice which contributes to lack of
appetite.

Considerable patience, tact and perseverance are all
required if the nurse is to succeed in persuading a deeply
depressed person to take food and fluids in adequate
amounts.

At mealtimes, the person's comfort is ensured by a
gentle reminder to visit the toilet before sitting down to
eat. A glass of water helps counteract dryness of the
mouth—a common unwanted effect of antidepressant
therapy. Small quantities of attractively served food of a
variety known to be preferred by the person are offered.
His primary nurse may need to find out from accompanying relatives during the admission procedure about
dietary preferences.

Supervision of the depressed person's food intake should not be interpreted by a new student to mean placing a plate of food in front of the person then going off to do something else, only returning from time to time to prompt him to eat or to comment on lack of progress, that the food will be getting cold. At mealtimes it may be necessary to draw up a chair alongside the person, if he has clearly shown that he has no wish to eat, and quietly conveying by words of encouragement, concern and an unhurried manner, that the nurse fully intends to remain until some nourishment is taken. Food supplements may replace one or more courses if appropriate.

Most people respond to this positive approach, though very occasionally the nurse may find it necessary initially to place the fork or spoon in the depressed person's hand to encourage him. Any successful nursing measure is recorded together with the amount taken.

Constipation may be associated with depression, and the effects of some antidepressants, lack of exercise and low fibre diet may all add to the problem. Laxatives are sometimes required and their effects often need to be monitored by the nurse.

To Re-establish Normal Sleep Patterns

Sleep is often disturbed in depression and any improvement in the person's sleep pattern may be taken as one of the earliest indices of the onset of improvement in mood. Complaints of late insomnia, that is, getting off to sleep but wakening early, then finding it impossible to get off again are often experienced by people who are depressed.

Early morning is a period of the day when the depressed person can find life quite intolerable (McKenzie,

1985). The night nurse may be able to engage him in some simple ward chore at this time to prevent his being totally immersed in morbid preoccupations, and by working alongside him she will be able to observe him the more closely.

Social Needs

In the early stages of a severely depressive disorder the person's social needs are few in number: 'it is useless to ask people who are beyond words . . . to look at themselves, at their relationships' ('Katy', 1985).

These words from someone who has experienced severe depression are a reminder to the nurse that the person's initial social needs are essentially at a very basic level. Regular and frequent contacts throughout the day with a member of the nursing team, or perhaps a close relative, will suffice to meet the deeply depressed person's need for the presence of another human being. Altschul (1985) comments that when she suffered from depression she found small talk and social conversation with a nurse, which 'was natural, unforced, never condescending, and which never seemed critical or derogatory' was much appreciated. The appropriate use of nonverbal communication in such situations has been alluded to earlier.

Gradually, as improvement occurs, the person may be persuaded to mix with one or two other people in a group. Once able to interact more confidently with fellow patients in this way, the support, warmth and friendship offered by them can be of enormous therapeutic value.

Increasing participation in activities organized by other members of the multidisciplinary care team, in addition to those available in the ward, provide further opportunities to satisfy the social needs of depressed people on their way to recovery.

CARE STUDY 3

In an earlier part of this chapter a description was given of how Mrs K was successfully cared for in the community when she had a depressive illness. Unfortunately two years after her last contact with the CPN she again became depressed. On this occasion Mrs K reluctantly agreed to be admitted to the local psychiatric unit of the general hospital, despite her firm conviction that nothing could be done for her, that she was not ill and that her current state of mind was entirely due to her past wickedness.

On admission Mrs K presented with a picture of deep depression. Movements and speech were slow and laboured; replies were monosyllabic and barely audible. She showed little or no interest in her new surroundings. Details about Mrs K's recent activities—or lack of them—were therefore given by accompanying relatives, her husband, Richard and daughter Jennie. It seemed that for the past week or so Mrs K had been increasingly reluctant to get out of bed in the morning and for most of the day she was apathetic, doing and saying little. Richard expressed particular concern over the fact she had been taking only very small amounts of food and drinking very much less than usual.

As well as information from relatives, data from the nursing assessment were compiled from nurses' observations of Mrs K made during the admission procedure and from subsequent interactions. It was decided that a formal interview with Mrs K would be postponed meantime in view of her inability to concentrate because of distress from her morbid thoughts.

Meanwhile it was determined that many of Mrs K's symptoms were similar to those experienced when depressed previously but much more severe on this occasion (see Care Study 1 above).

Furthermore, whereas during her earlier period of depression she had admitted to the CPN that she experienced feelings of guilt and unworthiness, this time Mrs K expressed a fixed false belief (delusion) that she had been wilfully unkind to her father prior to his death and that she had consistently neglected to visit him. It was also observed that Mrs K kept repeatedly searching through a collection of papers in her handbag 'to find proof' of her wrongdoings.

Jennie was visibly upset when she spoke to the nursing staff of the fact that her mother had on several occasions recently insisted she was a bother to her family and that it would be better for everyone if she were to die.

Using a modification of the human needs model of nursing Mrs K's immediate needs were identified from the initial nursing assessment, which focused on the difficulties Mrs K was experiencing in physical, psychological and social functioning due to her severely depressed mood.

While many of the needs and nursing interventions described earlier in relation to the general care of a person who is deeply depressed are also applicable to Mrs K's care, a selection of those of specific relevance to this care study are included as follows.

Physical needs:

1 To be cared for in a safe environment.
2 To be given an adequate intake of food and fluids.

Psychological and social needs:

1 To be given therapeutic responses to delusional talk.

2 To have self-esteem raised.

Though it was not until later when Mrs K's depressed mood had begun to lift and her needs were reassessed that she was able to take a substantive part in planning her care, it was vital meanwhile that a sensitive explanation was always given for all nursing interventions necessary to meet her needs. Richard and Jennie were also kept fully informed and in turn they supplied practical personal details such as Mrs K's dietary likes and dislikes, her hobbies and interests. Mrs K never ate eggs and did not take sugar in coffee or tea. Three days later Richard was delighted when asked if he could bring in a few photographs of their first grandchild, Neil, aged four months. Mrs K's primary nurse hoped to use them as a topic of conversation in the evenings when she had found Mrs K's mood to be slightly less depressed at that time of day.

To ensure Mrs K's safety needs were met, the risk category often known as 'close observation' was enforced. To know of Mrs K's whereabouts was necessary because of her preoccupation with morbid thoughts about what she felt to be the futility of living without any hope for the future.

At first Mrs K needed a lot of persuasion to take her prescribed medication (sertraline—see Appendix C): a member of the nursing staff remained with her to ensure it was swallowed since Mrs K was adamant that no amount of drugs could possibly help, that nothing was of any use.

Mealtimes were another occasion when Mrs K required to be given a great deal of encouragement and support. Despite the individual attention of her primary nurse, Mrs K took only tiny amounts of normal diet, however attractively served, and had to have fortified drinks to supplement her nutritional intake and prevent any further weight loss.

For several days following admission Mrs K's deeply

depressed mood was conspicuously worse in the morning. She was frequently to be found alone in an isolated corner of the smaller of the dayrooms, seated in a hunched posture with her hands covering her face. Looking back at this stage of her stay, Mrs K said that she found a nurse's presence particularly comforting and reassuring. She also added that she was grateful that no pressure was put on her at this time to take part in ward activities though she did appreciate the sensitive way in which regular invitations were given to join the others.

The delusion of wickedness held by Mrs K was a source of much of her mental torment. It also distressed her family who repeatedly assured nursing staff that in fact Mrs K had been a most devoted daughter, latterly giving up almost all of her limited free time to be with her father, confined to the house because of the severity of his arthritic disorder.

On one occasion during a handover session, a student on his mental health placement, knowing the facts of Mrs K's concern for her late father, admitted how difficult it was to resist the temptation to argue with Mrs K's delusional talk, rather than respond to her distress, though he was well aware this would be futile—and non-therapeutic. Ten days later, however, he was glad to have noted that Mrs K now seemed somewhat less convinced about her wickedness and had sought his reassurance with the words: '*You* don't think I'm an evil person do you? . . . these ideas are part of my illness aren't they?'

Nursing interventions to boost Mrs K's self-esteem—if only for a short spell at a time—seemed to have a positive outcome on at least two occasions. One evening Mrs K was surprised when her primary nurse asked if she could see some of her new grandson's photographs. Mrs K asked how the nurse knew of Neil's existence and was visibly moved to be told of the nurse's interest and concern. The photographs were then taken slowly from her handbag and though she said little it was clear Mrs K felt a glow of pride when the nurse commented favourably on Neil's appearance. The other occasion was two days later shortly before her visitors were due to arrive. Mrs K, after considerable persuasion, agreed to wear the new sweater and perfume Jennie had bought for her. It was noted that Mrs K held herself slightly more erect than usual as she greeted her family that afternoon. The first signs of a gradual improvement in Mrs K's mood were noted when she required somewhat less coaxing at mealtimes and one evening began to eat her supper without any prompting. The night nurse also reported that Mrs K was sleeping for longer periods rather than wakening at 2 a.m. as she had done during the early period of her stay. Ten days after admission Mrs K's primary nurse commented that the previous evening Mrs K had been prepared for the first time to concede that the day's activities had produced some positive thoughts and experiences for her, as opposed to her usual exclusively morbid and negative ones.

A multidisciplinary team approach to Mrs K's care was introduced on her sixth day in the unit. The occupational and the music therapist each talked with Mrs K and carried out an assessment of her potential for gaining benefit from attendance at their respective departments.

Initially Mrs K showed little enthusiasm for the idea of being involved in the activities offered though did agree to give them a try. After her attendances had become lengthier and more frequent, the occupational therapist reported to the multidisciplinary team meeting that Mrs K had shown more willingness to participate—especially in the relaxation sessions held each afternoon.

Towards the end of her third week in hospital a visit home was arranged at a meeting with Mrs K, her husband and the psychiatrist responsible for her medical care. This successful visit was followed a week later by an overnight stay. Several days before Mrs K's discharge the CPN who had known her two years earlier visited the unit and together agreed on a date for a follow-up appointment. Mrs K was also given a psychiatric outpatient appointment before she left hospital.

SUMMARY

It has been said that depression is difficult to understand for those who have never experienced it. Having made use in this chapter of hypothetical care studies and the actual words of people who have suffered from a depressive disorder it is hoped that this difficulty will have been at least partially overcome for the inexperienced learner. Some of the possible causes of depression have been explored followed by a discussion of the psychological, physical and social needs of the depressed person in the community. The second part of this chapter described the hospital-based care of the severely depressed sufferer and included the nursing interventions—in particular to meet the safety needs—of the person at risk of taking his own life.

REFERENCES

Altschul A (1985) There won't be a next time. In: Rippiere V & Williams R (eds) *Wounded Healers*. Chichester: Wiley and Sons.

Beck A (1976) *Cognitive Therapy and the Emotional Disorders*. New York: Penguin.

Brown GW & Harris TO (1978) *The Social Origins of Depression*. London: Tavistock.

Burton V (1991) Real nurses don't go mad. *Nursing Times* **87**(36): 50–51.

Gray E (1983) Severe depression: a patient's thoughts. *British Journal of Psychiatry* **143**: 319–322.

Henry J (ed.) (1988) *British Medical Association: Guide to Medicines and Drugs*. London: Dorling Kindersley.

Jehu D (1988) *Beyond Sexual Abuse: Therapy with Women who were Childhood Victims*. Chichester: Wiley.

'Katy' (1985) Learning to Live. In: Rippiere V & Williams R (eds) *Wounded Healers*. Chichester: Wiley.

Mackarness R (1976) *Not all in the Mind*. London: Pan Books.

McKenzie A (1985) Personal view. *British Journal of Medicine* **291**: 1044.

Murray Parkes C (1972) *Bereavement*. London: Penguin.

Peplau H (1952) *Interpersonal Relations in Nursing*. New York: Putman.

Salmons P (1984) Suicide in high buildings. *British Journal of Psychiatry* **145**: 469–472.

Smyth M & Craddock N (1989) Hospital suicide. *British Journal of Psychiatry* **154**: 728.

Winokur G (1981) *Depression: the Facts*. Oxford: Oxford University Press.

Chapter 8
Caring for the Person who is Elated and Overactive

INTRODUCTION

Marked elevation of mood and overactivity are part of the picture presented by a person who is showing what is known as manic behaviour which may be said to be on one side of a coin, with depression on the other. Alternatively one could place depression at one extremity of a mood scale and elation and overactivity at the opposite. Should a person exhibit manic behaviour (or hypomanic behaviour—a less acute form and one more commonly seen nowadays), having previously experienced a depressive illness, or vice versa, the terms manic–depressive psychosis or bipolar illness are often used. Other characteristics of a manic episode may include pressure of speech, disinhibition, delusions of grandeur, decreased need for sleep, distractibility and irritability.

This chapter continues with a graphic personal account by someone who has experienced some of the phenomena outlined above, followed by a description of nursing care required to meet the needs of the person who is elated and overactive and requires hospital admission. The second part of the chapter will look at community-based care. It will be noted that though an attempt has again been made to separate the patient's needs into three groups, i.e. psychological, physical and social, there is still considerable overlap among them. For example, the decision to include: 'To have limits set on disinhibited behaviour' under the heading of psychological needs of the person, rather than social, is quite arbitrary.

Howard (1988) who has suffered periods of depression and, less frequently, of mania over the past several years, describes the onset of the early changes which herald a manic phase and signify the need for immediate professional help:

> First, there are physical indications that all is not well. My heart feels as if it is beating faster. . . . I sleep less and wake up brimful of energy. My speech is more urgent. And then the mental agonies begin in the flights of fantasy.

Describing an earlier episode at a time when this sufferer was as yet unable to recognize the early warning signs, she elaborates further on the 'flights of fantasy':

> I felt elated, euphoric and thought that everything I touched would turn to gold. . . . At one stage I even believed I was the Virgin Mary reincarnated. My brain was travelling at a faster speed than the rest of me. I chattered non-stop. . . . I believed I was invincible.

HOSPITAL-BASED CARE

Identification of Needs and Nursing Interventions

Psychological Needs

To Have Disturbed Behaviour Responded to Empathetically

Empathetic responses to the person who is convinced it is possible to 'solve the world's problems in seven days, unite Ireland, feed starving people' (Gray, 1988) may include being available to listen attentively and patiently, without contradicting or arguing ineffectually and non-therapeutically (see also Chapter 7 for possible responses to delusional talk); every opportunity is taken to reinforce reality when interacting with this patient. Treating the overactive and elated person with sensitivity, respect and concern for his dignity and self-esteem, will help to foster the development of a trusting relationship. To assist the person to feel psychologically secure, the nurse has to make every effort to remain calm even when this is extremely difficult: the need for regular breaks when caring for the overactive person is very important. If the occasion arises it can be equally therapeutic for the patient if the nurse responds in a firm but gentle way to disturbed behaviour. A flexible approach is very important when trying to meet this person's ever-changing needs and endeavouring to respond appropriately to his unpredictable reactions.

To Have Limits Set on Disinhibited Behaviour

Therapeutic use is made of the overactive patient's short attention span and distractibility to prevent embarrassing situations arising from his disinhibited actions. For example, clothing may be a source of annoyance to the patient and the nurse's opportune intervention with a suggestion that they might go together to his room and find something lighter to wear can prevent the patient from undressing in a crowded dayroom.

This will ensure the person's dignity is preserved and he is protected from behaving in a way that would be acutely embarrassing for him to recall at a later date.

Sensitive explanations are given and opportunities are

found to discuss with the person the reasons for setting such limits on behaviour. Every episode of normal social behaviour should be positively reinforced.

Physical Needs

To Take an Adequate Intake of Food and Fluids

The overactive patient would seem to regard his basic physical needs as too mundane and time wasting to warrant his attention. He has more interesting plans in mind than stopping to eat, and is uninterested in taking enough food at a time when his energy requirements are increased due to his almost perpetual motion.

It may be less stimulating and distracting for the patient, and more peaceful for his fellow patients, if he can be gently coaxed to have meals in a quieter area of the unit, or in the privacy of his own room during the time when he is most disturbed. A full meal is seldom eaten: this would involve too long a period of unacceptable inactivity. To make sure his nutritional needs are met, the nurse can have nourishing sandwiches and high calorie drinks readily available to offer the patient at opportune moments during the day. A record should be kept of the amount taken.

Elimination needs can also be disregarded by the elated and overactive person who may be at risk of constipation from his medication. Careful monitoring is a necessary part of his plan of care.

To Keep Environmental Stimulation to a Minimum

To prevent the patient—already overstimulated as a result of his being hypomanic—from still further stimula-

tion and near physical exhaustion (a risk before the introduction of drugs such as haloperidol—see Appendix C)
nursing interventions which reduce environmental stimuli can be therapeutic. If possible, for example, the
patient might be cared for initially in a quiet area of the
unit. It is not realistic for the nursing staff to be able to do
more than try to reduce unnecessary stimulation but
sedentary activities, such as card games or looking at
magazines, however briefly, might afford a short, beneficial respite for both patient and staff.

The less acutely disturbed patient will benefit from a
structured programme of activities to suit his increased
energy levels, without allowing him to become overtired,
and to take into account his low boredom threshold.
Competitive games should be kept in reserve until the
hypomanic patient can function as a team member without totally disrupting the proceedings.

To Have Bathing and Dressing Supervised

It is likely that the elated and overactive person is much
'too busy' to attend to his hygiene needs, despite often
sweating a lot because of overactivity. Before tactfully
persuading him to have a bath or shower, the nurse may
find it helpful to adopt the strategy of having everything
required in readiness beforehand; otherwise the patient
may lose patience with what he perceives as undue
dilatoriness on the part of the nurse and dash off elsewhere. Left unsupervised the patient might 'escape'
from the shower and run along the corridor without any
clothes on. Sexual disinhibition can also be a feature of
this disorder and the female patient may appreciate,
later, attempts by the nursing staff to preserve her

dignity by offering subtle guidance when selecting suit-able clothes to wear in mixed company.

To be Cared For in a Safe Environment

To ensure the overactive person's safety and that of other patients an increased level of supervision is required in the acute stage of this condition.

Fellow patients may sometimes became exasperated to the point of threatening physical aggression if exposed to the manic patient's noisy, exuberant and sometimes argumentative behaviour for any length of time. Once again, by making use of the patient's distractibility, the nurse can quickly intervene to avert a potentially explosive situation.

The patient's unpredictable and impulsive behaviour together with a scant regard for personal safety requires close supervision by the nursing staff to anticipate and prevent hazards in the patient's immediate environment. For example, prompt drying up of the 'flooding' that often follows the manic patient's washing activities is necessary if accidents are to be avoided.

To Have Adequate Sleep

During the late evening the nurse has to think of measures to help the patient prepare for sleep. The elated and overactive patient will regard the idea of sleep as a waste of time and quite unnecessary. But if he can be per-suaded to have a warm, soothing bath it may help him 'unwind'. Once the patient is in bed the nurse's efforts to maintain a calm, non-stimulating environment may help him to remain there. Soft slow-tempo background music may help to provide a relaxed atmosphere conducive to sleep.

Social Needs

When the period of overactivity and disinhibited behaviour is most acute, it is particularly therapeutic for the patient to have a primary nurse or key worker assigned to his care. Too many new faces are a source of increased stimulation at a time when it is preferable to limit as much as possible the patient's social interactions. Visitors are best restricted to the person's immediate family. Despite honest and sensitive explanations, the patient lacking insight into his illness finds such measures totally unreasonable: when less disturbed he will be grateful as stated earlier, for having had his self-respect preserved and of there being fewer embarrassing incidents to repress.

The elated, overactive person can be very witty and highly amusing. His gaiety and good humour is often infectious, and he delights in an audience. It is impossible not to laugh *with* him sometimes, but the nurse can prevent the patient being laughed *at* when, for example, expressing delusions by quickly intervening and distracting the patient towards other activities. Similarly, this nursing skill is useful to avoid the patient's gregariousness interfering with fellow patients' privacy when visitors are present. This need to impose restrictions lessens immediately the first signs of improvement are noticed. The patient can then begin to be a more active participant in his plan of care and discuss with the nurse the need to establish what constitutes appropriate and inappropriate standards of behaviour. This will be helpful for the patient as he gradually regains his former self-control and ability to function normally.

CARING FOR THE PERSON WHO IS ELATED AND OVERACTIVE IN THE COMMUNITY

The signs and symptoms of elated and overactive behaviour will always manifest themselves first when the person is living at home in the community (unless the person is already in hospital). They may begin insidiously and not become problematic until the spouse or partner realizes that their joint bank account has become grossly overdrawn, or they become exhausted themselves from lack of sleep due to the sufferer's own overactivity. Manic-depressive psychosis is one of the major mental illnesses that can have a profound effect on the relatives and immediate family members who are exposed to the consequences of the hypomanic behaviour. It is important that they receive a swift response from the health services so that treatment can begin at the earliest signs. If the condition is allowed to progress too far it becomes increasingly difficult for the person to recognize that he is ill and in need of care; he continues to resist all attempts to treat the condition, until the only course left is for him to be admitted under a section of the Mental Health Act.

Manic-depressive psychosis is a condition of exaggerated mood swings, but it is also a condition that responds well to medication which lessens the degree of the mood swing. Many people who suffer from this condition are able to control their own symptoms with training and education about recognition of their symptoms. With the encouragement and cooperation of family members it is possible to minimize the more disturbing effects of the illness. CPNs, by building up good, trusting relationships with the sufferers and their families, can enable them to take the appropriate action in time to prevent an admission to hospital.

Lithium carbonate is a drug that is often used in the treatment of people with this disorder. It can, however, be highly toxic if there is too much present in the body so that careful monitoring is essential in the form of regular blood checks. These may be taken by the person's GP in the surgery or health centre. Some CPNs will do this, provided they have received phlebotomy training—the taking of blood—as this is considered an extended role of the nurse. Many services hold 'Lithium Clinics' where staff who have special expertise in this field see these people, assess their mental state, their medication, their lithium levels; give counselling and support as required, and, over the years, come to know these people very well and are able to recognize their mood swings quickly.

CPNs can play an important part in enabling people to return to their normal lives, following an acute episode of hypomania during which the sufferer may have caused embarrassment and even fear among families and neighbours. Sensitive discussion can allay fears and anxieties. Discussion with organizations such as the Citizens' Advice Bureau can help to sort out debts incurred while ill. Joining a local branch of the Manic-Depressives Association, where meeting with fellow-sufferers of the condition who offer support and helpful advice from their own experiences, can often be more meaningful to people than hearing the same from professionals.

SUMMARY

The care of the person who is elated and overactive presents a considerable challenge: flexibility of approach to keep up with swiftly changing needs, the timely use of distractibility and the importance of setting behavioural limits to avoid future embarrassment are some of the key skills required by an empathetic nursing staff.

From the foundation of a trusting relationship with the CPN, the person who is vulnerable to episodic elation and overactivity can become an active and knowledgeable partner in his care. Education, support and the monitoring of drug compliance by the CPN on a regular basis can often forestall hospital admission.

FURTHER READING

Ironbar N & Hooper A (1989) *Self-instruction in Mental Health Nursing*. London: Baillière Tindall.
Lyttle J (1986) *Mental Disorder*. London: Baillière Tindall.

REFERENCES

Gray P (1988) Dream or nightmare? *Nursing Times* **84**(48): 63–65.
Howard B (1988) Mania. *Openmind* **35**: 11.

Chapter 9
Caring for the Person who is Experiencing Hallucinations and Disordered Thinking

INTRODUCTION

People may experience hallucinations or disordered thinking when suffering a variety of conditions, but it is when these become a persistent feature of life and begin to interfere with normal daily activities or relationships and affect the way someone sees and relates to the world that they become the concern of psychiatrists and those working in the field of mental health. When these phenomena occur together in the absence of clouding of consciousness (which may denote an underlying physical condition), the term *schizophrenia* may be applied. (For a more detailed description of the clinical features of this major *psychotic* disorder see Appendix A.)

No-one knows the true causes of schizophrenia and there is no known pathological test to diagnose schizophrenia. There have been many theories advanced, from biological to environmental causation, and research continues to try to discover the cause of this most distressing and damaging form of mental illness. Studies carried out in a number of countries under the auspices of the World Health Organization (WHO) have shown that the disease occurs across the world and can affect 1 in 100 people (WHO, 1979; Sartorius *et al.*, 1986). At present, diagnosis depends on the observation of symptoms.

Research has found that, wherever possible, early identification of the onset of schizophrenia, followed by early intervention and treatment of the symptoms, accompanied by education and support to both the patient and the family, can often prevent the need to go into hospital and can minimize the development of a long-term career in the psychiatric services with frequent relapses and admissions to hospital.

Around one-third of all sufferers diagnosed as having a major mental illness usually recover and are unlikely to relapse for at least five years, if at all. Another third usually require follow-up and care for most of their lives, with the occasional relapse at times when they are most vulnerable and subject to stress, when they may need to be admitted to hospital for short periods. The last third may well be so affected by the disease that they need to be cared for in a hospital setting where they can receive the treatment they need within a safe and secure environment for much longer periods (Figure 9.1). This

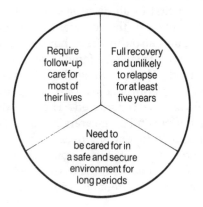

Fig. 9.1 Proportions of sufferers from major mental illness and the care they will require.

will usually be due to problems in controlling the symptoms sufficiently to enable the sufferer to live comfortably and at ease in the community.

Schizophrenia is an illness that is universal and not confined to any class, race, or age group. It can occur at any age but most frequently begins to manifest itself in young adulthood and not usually after the mid 50s. Children can appear to have had happy, normal years of development and to have performed well at school. Later they may begin to show signs of withdrawing from their friends, of not being able to sustain the standard of work they used to produce; their concentration begins to wane; they become suspicious of people, particularly those closest to them. Tensions can build up in the home, due entirely to a lack of understanding as to what is happening. Their perception of the world is changing. What was familiar is no longer to be trusted. It can be a terrifying and isolating experience, difficult for the person to describe without immediately being condemned as 'mad', with all that that implies.

This chapter first of all discusses some of the factors that contribute towards the occurrence and development of the disease and also the effect that the disease has on different areas of life such as families and relationships, studies and work. The special needs and requirements of people with schizophrenia who are living in the community will then be considered. The role of CPNs in working with them and their carers to encourage them to live as full and independent lives as possible will be explored. The last part of the chapter looks at hospital-centred care for people with the disease, whether this is in a short-stay setting, a rehabilitation setting, or a long-stay setting.

BIOLOGICAL FACTORS

There has been considerable research into the possibility of heredity as a factor in the causation of schizophrenia such as:

- the study of both identical and non-identical twins (Kringlen, 1987);
- the effect on the development of the disease in children born to parents with schizophrenia when they are adopted by parents without schizophrenia (Heston, 1966);
- brain imaging studies to discover whether there is physiological evidence for the disease;
- chromosome studies to try to identify which gene or genes may be responsible for the disease (Shelton & Weinberger, 1986).

From the body of all this research it is becoming clearer that there is an hereditary link, with a greater tendency to develop the disease if there is someone else in the family who has had it, but there is simply not enough knowledge yet to be able to claim with any certainty that schizophrenia is due to biological factors on their own.

ENVIRONMENTAL FACTORS

Whatever, eventually, the cause of schizophrenia may be discovered to be, research has established that the occurrence of relapse in the disease is related to the degree of stress experienced by the sufferer. This may be either stress caused by a sudden change or life-event, or a continual state of stress caused by living in a tense or highly charged environment. Research into 'expressed emotion' in families with a member suffering from schizophrenia has indicated that where there is a tendency to be over-critical, hostile and rejecting, over-involved or too intense and over-protective of the sufferer, the likelihood of relapse increases. If, however, relatives can be warm, accepting, non-critical and encouraging, the likelihood of relapse is reduced (Leff & Vaughn, 1985). Sufferers and families need to understand that full recovery may take a very long time, anything up to two years, during which time sufferers may well be able to return to work, return to their studies, and to pick up the friendships and relationships they had before their illness.

Other factors that are known to lead to successful recovery and prevent relapse include the following:

- continuing to take medication;
- education of both sufferer and relatives about schizophrenia;
- helping families to solve problems;
- improving their own communication;
- dealing with their criticism and over involvement;
- reducing contact between sufferer and relatives;
- e.g. attending a day hospital or day centre
- increasing social networks for both sufferer and the family;
- lowering expectations.

EFFECTS OF SCHIZOPHRENIA

Effect on the family

Families in which there is a member who has developed a schizophrenic illness may have experienced either a slow progression of withdrawal and dislocation or a sudden inexplicable eruption of odd behaviour and incomprehensible conversation. Parents and siblings may be affected in different ways. Individuals may feel responsible and involved or wish to dissociate themselves from what is happening within the family. Frequently, family members feel themselves becoming isolated from their previous social networks; they feel unable to go on holidays because they may feel embarrassed by the behaviour of the schizophrenic person. They find that the strain and anxiety of living with someone with a schizophrenic illness affects their own physical and mental health. Often there are financial implications arising from a member of the family living on social benefits or invalidity benefit which brings financial hardship and prevents the return to a fulfilling, active life. In some instances, family members prefer to cut themselves off from having any contact with the individual, or they minimize contact with families where the affected person is living. Families become broken up and lose the close ties and the support that comes with closeness, creating even greater isolation and distress and an increase in the 'burden of care'.

The National Schizophrenia Fellowship (1974, 1975) has been saying for many years that families have been left to shoulder the greatest amount of the caring for people discharged from hospital with schizophrenic conditions with very little support or preparation for coping. Community psychiatric nurses had begun to try to offer support and guidance to families, but it is through the pioneering work of community psychiatrists, psychologists, nurses and others who have researched into ways of working actively with families, that progress has been made in helping families to understand better the processes that contribute to relapse and breakdown. Talking with families and teaching them about the condition, its possible causes, the symptoms that occur with the disease, and the effect that these have on the sufferer, can all help greatly in changing the attitude of family members to the sufferer. It may then become easier for relatives to begin to consider different ways of behaving towards the sufferer which could minimize the recurrence of symptoms and relapse. Through working together with the family and the sufferer, these researchers have been able to develop programmes and approaches to care which enable both the sufferer and the relatives to recognize early signs and take sensible steps that are acceptable to all to prevent further relapse.

Effect of Schizophrenia on Academic Studies

Often the illness first begins to manifest itself when young people are preparing themselves for their adulthood. They are concentrating on passing exams, entering higher education, looking to start training and developing skills on which will depend the success of their future career. Expectations may have been set unrealistically high by both the person who develops the illness and by other family members. This is a stressful time for any young person and at present there is no adequate explanation for why any one member of a family may develop a schizophrenic illness rather than another. A significant number of young people who do develop the illness do so in the early years in higher education. Some are able to return and complete their studies, some may wish to but find that the effects of the illness, combined with the side-effects of the medication that they require in order to remain symptom-free, prevent them from being able to continue. This is a time when both the individual and the family need much help and encouragement to cope with their disappointment and to adjust to a different level of aspiration, one in which the individual can feel useful and fulfilled.

Effect of Schizophrenia on Job Prospects

A number of people with schizophrenic conditions will be able to hold jobs in the open market and lead reasonably normal lives, but there will be those who find the pressures of the wider world too stressful. These people may well be able to function quite adequately and productively in a more sheltered environment where there is an understanding of the difficulties that accompany the type of disability from which they suffer. Sheltered workshops provide just such an environment. There is an expectation that people attending should observe the same sort of discipline that is required of anyone in employment, such as arriving on time, working hard while at work, not being disruptive and wasting time, so that people feel they are respected for what they can achieve and are encouraged to do the best they can. In return they earn wages within the limits of the social security system, in addition to receiving whatever level of benefit to which they are entitled.

Effect of Schizophrenia on Relationships

One of the areas of life that often becomes particularly affected by the illness is that of relationships. To begin with, sufferers withdraw from family and friends who themselves may not recognize or understand what is happening. Some may feel rejected or embarrassed and give up trying to maintain the friendship. It is vitally important that relationships and friendships are not lost; that people are helped to understand what is going on and to see how they can play a crucial part in keeping the person suffering from this illness from becoming too detached from the real world. Community psychiatric nurses and all those who work in the mental health field have an important role in teaching and helping people, family members and friends, to learn how to understand and cope with living with someone with a long-term mental illness.

CARING FOR THE PERSON WITH HALLUCINATIONS AND DISORDERED THINKING IN THE COMMUNITY

People suffering from schizophrenia have a multiplicity of needs if they are to be able to live to the best of their ability, fulfilling their potential and enjoying all the facilities that most people enjoy. Nurses have an important role to play, alongside their professional colleagues and in collaboration both with other agencies from the statutory services, such as social services and primary care teams, and with voluntary organizations, such as MIND (The National Association for Mental Health), SAMH (The Scottish Association for Mental Health) and NSF (The National Schizophrenia Fellowship).

Community psychiatric nurses, when they receive referrals to take on the care of someone suffering from a schizophrenic illness, will usually adopt a problem-solving approach based on the nursing process (see Chapter 4).

- They will *assess* the needs of the individual, taking into account the psychological, physical and social needs and will involve the person and the immediate carers whenever possible.
- Once the CPNs have gathered as much information as possible, together with the person and the carers, they will jointly *plan* a programme of care, or agree a *care plan*, with both short-term and long-term goals.
- The next stage is to *implement* the care programme in order to achieve the goals set and agreed. These goals may involve the cooperation of other agencies, and it is one of the roles of the CPN to coordinate the different activities of each client and to liaise with the people concerned.
- The CPN will *evaluate* progress at all stages but it is particularly useful to set regular dates and times for a full evaluation of the care programme, at which all those who are involved with the care of each person can speak freely and honestly. Together they can review the work of the previous period, acknowledge successes and agree a new care programme with new goals. These may include some of the original goals which continue to be pertinent and include new areas which may help the individual to improve the quality of life they wish to lead.

The different needs of two groups of people will now be considered:

1 those who have suffered from the disease for many years and have been resettled into the community;
2 those who are newly diagnosed.

Rehabilitation/Resettlement of People with Long-standing Schizophrenic Illness

People may have been in hospital for long periods of their life, either because their families were unable or unwilling to have them back at home, or because their illness was such that they needed full-time care, or because there was not appropriate accommodation available for them outside hospital with enough resources to provide the type and amount of aftercare needed.

Most of this group of people who remain in hospital today do not really need to be living in a hospital. They could be cared for in a house or hostel in the community where there is properly trained and adequate staffing to make sure that they look after themselves and observe the basic activities of daily living (see pp. 71 and 184–8 for details of these activities).

There needs to be a whole range of sheltered accommodation available to choose from for these people, depending on their degree of ability and wish for more or less independence. Voluntary organizations such as MIND, the NSF, the Richmond Fellowship, the Mental Health Foundation and others have been providing sheltered accommodation for this group for many years. Housing associations and societies have become much more active since government legislation has encouraged funding to go to them to develop special needs housing for particular groups.

This range should include:

- 24 hour staffed hostels for the more disabled who require a greater amount of help and supervision;
- half-way houses for those who need to test out for themselves how well they can manage and to prepare themselves for greater independence;

- group homes for those who prefer to live with some company;
- supported bedsits for those who like more independence but recognize their own vulnerability and cope better if they have ready access to someone whom they can call upon if they feel themselves becoming unwell.

With encouragement and the opportunity to experiment with different levels of supervision many of this group of people are able to move into their own independent flats. They will probably always require a certain amount of support and follow-up care, but with the availability of properly planned daycare facilities, social and leisure time activities, regular monitoring and review of their mental health and abilities to manage their lives through contact with their GP and mental health team, there is no reason why this group should ever have to return to hospital life again.

Having appropriately supported accommodation in the community is not enough on its own. Although there has been much criticism directed at the traditional way in which people with long-term mental illnesses have been kept in hospitals, depriving them of the choice and freedom that the rest of society enjoys, the life and relationships built up within the community of the hospital had their own importance and relevance. Activity centres, industrial workshops, hospital farms and gardens provided some of the daytime activity for the residents. Social activities such as bingo evenings, sports activities and outings were organized on a regular basis. Friendships and romances were developed among the residents.

It has been found that when many of this group of long-term residents were resettled into the community, the quality of their lives, in fact, was reduced. They were no longer so easily able to keep up their old relationships; the same number of planned outings and activities were no longer available to them; there were too few similar facilities available to them in the community. It is hardly surprising that they became even more lonely, isolated and lost. The opportunity for choice may have been theirs, but the ability to take advantage of that choice was not theirs as they did not know how to choose.

Much more attention is *now* being given to the needs of people with long-term mental illness who have been resettled into the community. There are, for example:

- day centres, which provide a number of functions such as a 'drop-in' facility where people can, literally, drop in for a cup of tea, a chat, a game of darts or draughts, or to ask for advice or guidance on a problem;
- day hospitals, which can provide the focus for treatment, outpatient clinics, counselling;
- Community Mental Health Centres, which can be both the base from which Community Mental Health Teams operate and the centre to which people come for activity and company during the day or evening.

The Importance of Medication in Caring for People with Hallucinations and Disordered Thinking in the Community

Although the causes of schizophrenia are still unknown it is well established that neuroleptic drugs (see p. 342) do help to control the symptoms of the illness that interfere so much with leading an ordinary life:

- hallucinations that distort the sensory perceptions of the world;

- delusions to believe all manner of things that do not exist for the majority of people;
- disorders in thought processes that prevent communication with other people.

The drugs that are currently available are extremely potent and although they certainly do help to control symptoms they also, unfortunately, have a number of unpleasant side-effects that can interfere with other functions of the body. (See Appendix C for details of side-effects.)

As has already been discussed in Chapter 3, one of the clinical roles of the CPN is to monitor the effect of medication on the mental and physical state of each person. This is particularly important with those who have a major psychiatric disorder, as it is the combination of appropriate medication along with adequate social support and care that will ensure a successful adaptation to life in the community and reduce the need to return to hospital.

CARE STUDY 1

Mr Bill W has been in hospital for many years. He was admitted under a section of the Mental Health Act 1959, having caused his family much anxiety and distress over the previous years. Bill was slow to respond to treatment and the family had eventually refused to have Bill home again. As there was no suitable alternative accommodation available at that time Bill had remained in hospital. Over the years his mental state had settled, partly due to him receiving regular medication. Recently, he has been participating in a rehabilitation programme to enable him to be discharged into a sheltered hostel, managed by a local housing association. (For an example of the type of rehabilitation programme Bill might take part in, see pp. 183–8.) All those who are to be involved in caring for him as he adjusts to a new life in the community are present at a pre-discharge meeting. As well as this being good practice it is a requirement under the Care Programme Approach for anyone who has been in hospital for longer than six months (see Chapter 3).

These people include:

- Bill himself.
- The consultant psychiatrist who will continue to be responsible for his psychiatric care.
- The GP who will take on the responsibility for Bill's general medical care and who will be prescribing his medication.
- The CPN who will be coordinating the care programme for Bill and who will visit him on a regular basis.
- The primary nurse/key worker who has been working with Bill throughout his rehabilitation programme and who will continue to give him support and encouragement until he is settled.
- The occupational therapist (OT) who will be Bill's key worker at the day centre which he attends for three days a week.
- The manager of the sheltered workshop which Bill will start to attend for the other two days of the week.
- The warden of the sheltered hostel to which Bill will be moving.
- The social worker who is to try to locate Bill's children and re-establish links with his family.

All these people have a part to contribute to the ease and success with which Bill reintegrates into a new life in the community.

Decisions reached at the pre-discharge meeting:

- A date and time are agreed for Bill to begin a trial period in the hostel.
- In the meantime, he will continue to attend the day centre and start to attend the sheltered workshop so that he has a routine to follow.
- The primary nurse will accompany him for the first few days until he is confident and familiar with the journey to the workshop.
- The CPN will visit him regularly on the ward so that they can begin to know one another and build up a trusting relationship, as it is the CPN who will take over from the primary nurse as Bill becomes more settled outside hospital.
- The hostel warden will arrange for Bill to visit on several occasions so that he meets the other residents and will not feel quite so strange and alone when he moves in. Bill will need to know his way around his new locality and where to cash his benefit cheque; the warden will explain the intricacies of the housing benefit system.
- The consultant psychiatrist will see Bill in the outpatient clinic two weeks into his trial period to monitor how he is coping with the stress of a major life-event such as moving out of hospital after many years.
- The CPN will take him to meet the GP in his surgery during this time so that he knows where to go and is familiar with the protocol of going to see a GP.
- Finally, a date and time is agreed when Bill and all those present will meet again to review Bill's progress, to assess his needs in the light of his resettlement in the hostel, and to agree a new care programme with additional goals and targets.

This process will continue for as long as Bill and those concerned for his health and well-being believe it to be necessary, with the CPN as the central coordinating figure.

The role of the CPN in this situation is chiefly that of the care coordinator. There are many other people, all with a crucial part to contribute to the success of Bill's rehabilitation. It would be easy for some to contradict the efforts of the others quite unintentionally if they did not all know just what was needed for Bill. By arranging regular review meetings, at first more frequently as Bill starts his new life out of hospital, the CPN can ensure that things progress as smoothly as possible. By working together as a team, any signs of relapse can be picked up quickly, action can be taken early and unnecessay readmission to hospital can be avoided.

The Person Newly Diagnosed

People who have only recently developed the disease are no longer expected to spend many years in hospital. The aim nowadays is to prevent 'institutionalization' from developing, to try to keep people in touch with the real world from the moment of admission. Contact with family and friends is encouraged so that relationships are not lost, and interests are maintained. Care programmes are negotiated with the person which incorporate the usual living skills as illustrated in Bill's experience. However, it will always be necessary to remember the dangers of over-stimulation; too much pressure too soon can prevent progress both in hospital and in the community.

One of the main differences between this group and the previous group is that the illness can be difficult to stabilize in the early years and it may take time to find just the right combination of medication and activity and support for each individual. This may involve relapse and return of acute symptoms. It is during this period in particular that good care coordination and good liaison between all agencies, including the family, must be developed and maintained. Professional help and support must be available as quickly as possible to respond to carers, whether they be the family or those working in sheltered accommodation, so that readmission to hospital can be avoided or accessed depending on the degree of illness of each person.

Although the emphasis nowadays is on keeping episodes in hospital to a minimum, and plans for discharge and aftercare needs following discharge are encouraged from the start. Recovery from and learning to live with the condition of schizophrenia can take a long time and continues after discharge for many years.

CARE STUDY 2

Jenny S is 19 years old. She has recently been in hospital after suffering an acute psychotic episode (see Appendix A). She was an undergraduate student at university reading for an honours degree in history and sociology. She had been a bright student at school, good at games and a lively member of the school's drama group; she had had many friends. She is the third child of four in the family, two elder brothers and a younger sister. Her father is a successful teacher, being head of his department; her mother is a music teacher with a high reputation of achievement among her pupils. She is an emotional woman, noisy and flamboyant, quick to react and irritated by her husband's more methodical and prosaic nature. Consequently, there are many discussions that end in arguments and drama. All the family are bright and like to state their opinions, and, in spite of all the noise and tension that arises from this, they are a warm and united family. None of them can understand what has happened to Jenny or what can possibly have caused her to become so ill. She has been advised to take the rest of the academic year out and plan to return at the start of the next year. This gives her six months to recover and to stabilize on her medication.

While Jenny was in hospital (see pp. 179–83 for a description of inpatient care) it became apparent that she was able to upset her mother very easily and that her father seemed to cope with the whole situation by appearing indifferent and expecting Jenny to 'snap out of her funny ideas' in due course. It was agreed by the mental health team that the CPN, who had a particular interest and some training in working with families with a member suffering from schizophrenia, should visit and try to help the family understand more about the illness itself and learn how they could best help Jenny and themselves live with this knowledge. The CPN and a psychologist run a series of weekly groups consisting of six sessions of two hours' duration, for relatives who have a recently diagnosed member of the family with schizophrenia, where people can come and both learn more of the facts of the disease and give and gain support from other people who are also having to come to terms with a new situation in their lives. The plan is for the CPN to assess the family at home, and if appropriate, offer them the opportunity to attend the next course. In the meantime, the CPN will begin the more sensitive work of helping the family to recognize how, perhaps, living in a highly charged atmosphere all her life, plus all the stress of leaving home, coping with a strenuous academic programme and adjusting to all the new experiences and opportunities that life at a university offers, may well have contributed to her breakdown.

The other area of major concern with which they will all need support is encouraging Jenny to persevere with her medication. Jenny is on a depot injection which she receives fortnightly from the CPN. She is aware that her concentration level is not good. She has difficulty in focusing when reading and cannot remember what she has been reading. This clearly affects her ability to study. The CPN can support her through this early period and help her not to be too discouraged by slow progress. As the family are such high achievers with high expectations of their own success they will all need to learn how not to place too much pressure on Jenny and at the same time not to give up on her. Those aspects of the illness that are referred to as the 'negative symptoms' are often what families find the most difficult to understand and with which to live: loss of motivation, loss of emotion, social withdrawal. She will need space and time to allow healing to take place. The family will need time and support to understand this. It may be helpful to put them in touch with the local branch of the National Schizophrenia Fellowship whose aims are to provide support and education to sufferers of schizophrenia and to their carers.

The role of the CPN in this scenario is more specific than in the previous care study. With Jenny and her family, who illustrate the high expressed emotion discussed earlier, the CPN has an educative role and a supportive role arising from it. The CPN continues to work with Jenny on the care programme agreed while in hospital in order to prevent the loss of skills which occurred with Bill's experience. The clinical role involves, in Jenny's case, the administering of a depot injection, and the monitoring of both its effectiveness and any side-effects. Jenny and her family will need to know why the medication is necessary, what common side-effects occur, how to cope with them, when to see a doctor, how to recognize her own symptomatology, when to avoid triggers that lead to greater stress, and much more. Together, the CPN, Jenny and the family will become partners in Jenny's care, sharing the worries and anxieties, responding as and when necessary. The CPN will work closely with the rest of

the team, liaising and giving up-to-date progress reports.
The CPN will most certainly receive supervision for the
family work, as the dynamics and interplay of relationships
in such a situation will be complex and sensitive.

HOSPITAL-CENTRED CARE FOR THE PERSON EXPERIENCING HALLUCINATIONS AND DISORDERED THINKING

In hospital a combination of skilled nursing care, the contribution from other members of the multidisciplinary
team, and the appropriate medication, will usually effect
a favourable outcome for the newly diagnosed person
with an acute episode of schizophrenia. As was the case
with Jenny they can often then leave hospital after a relatively short stay.

This was not always so: in the past a substantial number
of people did not respond sufficiently to allow for early
discharge, and had to be transferred to a non-acute unit.
However, over the past four decades many people—
indeed more than half of the longer-stay population—
have, as we saw earlier with Bill, been able to move from
hospital to community after a period of rehabilitation. The
reasons for these discharges are varied. Factors include
changes in the management of hospitalized psychiatric
patients which began in the immediate post-war period
and were epitomized by the 'revolution in social psychiatry' (Warner, 1985)—a movement which owes much to
Maxwell Jones at Dingleton Hospital in Melrose and to
David Clark at Fulbourn. The introduction of social
psychiatry heralded the 'radical' notion of patients' participation in their own management; a practice now
widely accepted as an integral part of planning care.

Another important change was the advent in the mid-1950s of antipsychotic drugs, followed in the next decade by the start of successful rehabilitation programmes to prepare long-stay residents with potential for discharge to live outside hospital. In this section the care of people in three different care settings will be considered:

1 Short-stay
2 Non-acute/rehabilitation
3 Long-stay/sheltered

Care of the Person in a Short-stay Setting: Identification of Needs and Nursing Interventions

Psychological Needs

To be kept in touch with reality. The acutely disturbed person with hallucinations and thought disorder often shows a tendency to withdraw from social interaction, and according to Farr (1982), will 'drift from reality' if allowed to remain on one's own for long periods, becoming preoccupied with an inner, often terrifying, world. She goes on in her personal account to describe how the nurse's presence and meaningful conversation represented and reinforced reality for her. An important goal, although a difficult one to achieve at first for the less experienced nurse, is to establish contact and rapport with the withdrawn person in the hope of building a trusting nurse–patient relationship. Conversation can be largely one-sided in the early days following admission, with little or no positive feedback from the patient ('sometimes I didn't talk for days'; Farr, 1982). This can be a frustrating and uncomfortable experience for the new nurse; she will require help from experienced nursing staff to cope with these feelings. Their support and encouragement will allow her to persevere in her efforts to gain the person's trust.

Patient–nurse interactions should be regular, frequent and initially of short duration until the person gets accustomed to the nurse's presence. Reiterating these points, Farr also states that when the nurse was able to spend time with her and was patient with her, she gradually became more oriented to reality and more able to converse. Close observation of the patient's non-verbal cues may provide the nurse with a sensitive index of how long she should remain at any given time. Before leaving, the nurse may tell the patient when she intends to return. If subsequently, however, she finds herself unable to keep her promise, an explanation should be passed on to the patient. It would be all too easy for the inexperienced nurse to assume, wrongly, that this patient had probably not registered what she had said on the basis of a lack of any outward response on the patient's part.

Farr (1982) gives details in the personal account quoted above of the terror experienced by hearing 'voices' and of how comforting it was to have a nurse come into the room, be reminded by her that she was in hospital and reassured that all was well and that nothing extraordinary was in fact taking place around her.

In another personal account Hiles (1984) tells of her 'voice' informing her that she would have to have her head chopped off, then lie in a coffin until 'he' came back to sew it on again for her.

A person who is disturbed by auditory hallucinations such as those described above may be comforted by the nurse stating that she intends to stay with her (or him) while the distress lasts. The nurse may also wish to add that she is, however, unable to 'hear' this person's 'voices', while nevertheless conveying, by her continued presence, an understanding to the patient of how frightening such an experience must be.

To experience fewer distressing auditory hallucinations. It is important for the nurse to be aware that 'voices' tend to be more troublesome for the person if sensory input is reduced, and that social stimulation in the form of encouragement to listen to meaningful speech during a one-to-one nurse–patient interaction has a beneficial influence in controlling auditory hallucinations (Margo *et al.*, 1981).

Work by Cutting (1989) points out that incidents which create states of tension or arouse the patient's anger exacerbate hallucinatory experiences. If the nurse is aware of this she can try to anticipate and avert such incidents whenever possible.

Close observation of acutely disturbed patients is also necessary since they may behave impulsively and unpredictably in response to an auditory hallucination and be at risk of harming themselves or others. Robinson (1984) recalls a patient who burnt his wrist with a cigarette because a famous pop star 'told' him to do so. Prompt intervention by the nursing staff can defuse tense situations which may also arise from the patient's disturbed (delusional) thinking: for example, a fellow patient, who is repeatedly being falsely accused by a deluded patient of hatching malicious plots against him, may be provoked into threats of physical aggression. (See p. 131 above for suggested verbal responses to the person's disordered (e.g. delusional) thinking.)

Physical Needs

To be prompted to attend to self-care. Self-care in the context of this chapter is defined as the ability of the person with long-term needs to care for personal hygiene, appearance etc. (See p. 66 for a more comprehensive definition.) Patients' disordered thinking may lead to self-neglect. They may not take the initiative to care for their personal hygiene and will require to be gently reminded to do so. For one patient, bathing was a welcome occasion to wash away his 'evil thoughts' but on the other hand he did not appreciate the need to change his underwear regularly due to his thoughts being disturbed.

To be encouraged to take adequate nourishment. Individuals who are extremely withdrawn and acutely hallucinated may have to be approached by the nurse and invited to come to the dining room at mealtimes, otherwise they may remain in their rooms unmindful of the need for food and drink. Furthermore, there are sometimes those who hear a 'voice' telling them their food is being poisoned or adulterated and refuse to eat unless allowed to prepare and cook their own food. However, with skilled nursing care and appropriate medication such a solution may be needed only for a very short period of time.

Social Needs

As soon as the person who is experiencing hallucinations and disordered thinking begins to relate more comfortably to a nurse, for example his primary nurse, his care plan will then focus more on meeting social needs, with if possible the patient and the nurse agreeing on the short-term goals to be achieved. At first the patient, with the nurse providing the necessary support and encouragement, may feel able to join a small social group for a limited period of time, then gradually a programme of selected activities can follow, the aim being to reduce the time the disturbed individual spends isolated from others.

Unlike Jenny some people have had a long history of social withdrawal going back a number of years prior to coming into hospital for the first time. After a social skills assessment has identified strengths and weaknesses in social functioning, the person may be willing to join a social skills group to help improve quality of life after discharge (see also pp. 278–83).

Care of the Person in a Rehabilitation Setting

Reassessment of the person with longer-term needs

Before participating in an active rehabilitation programme (see below) people who have been in hospital for some time often need to be reassessed to identify again their individual needs. If these needs can be met successfully then, as happened with Bill, discharge into a community setting may be arranged.

(Re)assessment is also necessary to consider an individual's strengths and how these can be further developed. There are a number of standard assessment tools used in rehabilitation units: the Morningside (a district of Edinburgh) Rehabilitation Status Scale (Affleck & McGuire, 1984) is an example of a large scale assessment carried out by nursing staff. It is also useful to monitor progress at the end of each stage in a person's rehabilitation programme.

Identification of Needs and Interventions

To participate in an active rehabilitation programme. From the (re)assessment data, often collected over a period of time, a programme specially devised for each person is drawn up.

Any discussion of the programme and goals to be met must include the active and voluntary participation of the person involved. Short-term goals must be realistic and negotiable: the long-term goal of ultimate transfer to the community should not be seen in such a way that the person feels pressurized, with any setback interpreted as failure. Setbacks, if and when they do arise, should be considered rather as normal occurrences of little account in the longer term: emphasis is placed on success—however tentative in the early stages. Regular reassessment and evaluation of progress become an integral part of the programme and detailed feedback sessions take place between each resident and a member of the nursing team.

Nurses, and other members of the multidisciplinary team, must always avoid expecting the resident to proceed at too rapid a pace. Their hopes—and disappointments—inadvertently conveyed to the resident, can quickly raise anxiety levels. The recurrence of disturbed behaviour, episodes of depression and even suicide have been recorded in those who have felt the expectations of others to be overwhelming and unrealistic.

The fear of premature discharge is also sometimes a cause for concern to residents. They must know they are free to opt out of the programme at any time, temporarily or permanently, if they wish. Ideally each person is allocated a primary nurse (or key worker—a term commonly used in this setting), someone they rely on to give encouragement and support and with whom they can build a relationship.

To (re)learn or improve on a variety of skills. Included in the rehabilitation programme will be the skills the person requires to learn, re-establish or improve before embarking on a new life outside hospital. Some examples are:

(i) Initiating self-care. The ability to care adequately for personal hygiene and also to dress appropriately have been included in the important skills needed for successful adjustment to community life (Barker, 1985). The skills required to care for clothes, such as being able to use a washing machine and an iron, are likely to have to be learnt by the male resident and re-established by his female counterpart.

(ii) Looking after one's living environment. The skills involved in routine housekeeping duties, washing-up, dusting etc., cannot be regarded as being of concern only to women. It is not unusual for a small number of men to live together in a group home on discharge from hospital and to do all the domestic chores without female help.

Teaching such skills, however, calls for the nurse to make maximum use of her sense of humour. She can then turn an otherwise tedious and dreary task for the learners into a light-hearted occasion, while her active participation in the work to be done allows the opportunity for social interaction with the residents.

(iii) Preparing and cooking meals. The nursing staff, and also the occupational therapist, as a member of the rehabilitation team, play key roles in teaching people the skills involved in preparing and cooking food. Practices vary: the ward kitchen may be used or the larger fully equipped facility in the occupational therapy department may be chosen, especially for those who are in need of more intensive tuition. As confidence is gained, cooking Sunday lunch for fellow residents may be used as a practice session. Included in the teaching sessions is an emphasis on the need for food hygiene and safety standards to be closely adhered to during the preparation and cooking of food.

Furthermore, in settings where residents and staff sit down to eat together, use can be made of this excellent opportunity for residents to improve their level of social functioning.

(iv) Self-administering medication. Self-administration of drugs can present problems at first for this group of people who hitherto have had almost no occasion to think about when, and how much, and what type of medication to take. Time is set aside to help the person appreciate the need to take medication regularly. It should be seen as an extremely important part of the rehabilitation programme. Failure to comply with drug regimens after discharge is a not infrequent reason for readmission.

A special medicines trolley equipped with small individual compartments, containing perhaps one week's supply of drugs, may be used for the purpose of teaching self-administration. Initially a certain amount of prompting and supervision by the resident's primary nurse or key worker is necessary until there is competence in this particular skill. Indeed some people continue to have difficulty with medication after they leave hospital and a considerable amount of supervision by relatives or the CPN is necessary to ensure success.

(v) Interacting socially. Although opinion is divided, there are a number of authorities who contend that the interpersonal difficulties experienced by people in longer-term inpatient facilities are based in part on a paucity of social skills. These practitioners affirm that a training programme directed towards improving the person's level of social functioning yields a number of beneficial results, not least of these being a more successful adjustment to living in the community for those for whom discharge from hospital is a possibility at some future date.

Specific measurements used to assess an individual's level of social functioning include the use of a questionnaire to be completed by the resident (Barker, 1985); or a social skills rating scale is completed by the nurse in order to compile a profile of the person's level of competency in such non-verbal features of interpersonal behaviour as eye contact, facial expression and posture (Trower *et al.*, 1978).

In the first group session of a social skills training programme the focus may be on the need to improve basic conversational skills; at a later date activities using role-play and video recordings, as, for example, in assertiveness training—often an integral part of the training programme—make up some of the sessions.

However, the nursing team are ideally placed not only to act as group facilitators but to grasp every opportunity throughout the day to aid the resident to generalize newly found social skills.

Remedial drama and group discussion techniques have also been used as treatment procedures to improve social competency but neither has been found to be as effective as social skills training programmes.

(vi) Pursuing new interests and hobbies. Ideally, through regular contact with the occupational and work therapists, many people who have been in hospital for some time will gradually have been able to re-establish, or learn new skills of value when seeking future employment. For example, many hospitals have facilities where residents can learn computing skills if they so wish. But, in reality, it can often be very difficult for ex-psychiatric patients to find work, particularly in times of high unemployment, notwithstanding the substantial numbers of employers, for example local industrialists, who are sympathetic to the plight of this group of people and who do make a very worthwhile contribution to the provision of employment opportunities.

In the light of this problem, members of the rehabilitation team such as the art, drama, music and recreational therapists, use their expertise to encourage the individual to cultivate new interests and hobbies that he can continue to pursue in the community.

Despite these strenuous efforts, Macauley (1989) cites the results of a questionnaire, completed by a group of ex-patients living in the community, which show a lack of social activities to be the main problem facing them in their day-to-day living. He goes on to describe a club based in a local community high school as one remedy for combating this social isolation. Staffed by local hospital personnel, the school's community education worker and several of the staff from the school, this club affords attenders opportunities not only to socialize but also to participate in sporting and educational activities.

The resultant increased awareness of mental health problems among the staff and students at the high school is considered to be an extremely important by-product of the club, and students from the school have begun to visit the local psychiatric hospital on a regular basis.

(vii) Being able to budget successfully. The skills needed to budget successfully on what is often a modest income can be difficult to learn, or relearn if the resident has been in hospital for many years; many people have forgotten, for example, the need to set priorities when trying to manage on a limited income. Despite having the intricacies of statutory benefits explained to him, the newly discharged person may still find himself in financial difficulties due to non-payment of bills. The CPN, with the person's consent, may be able to help by arranging for monies to be deducted at source to prevent vital services being cut off.

Moving into the Community

As illustrated in Bill's care study, the success of effecting the smooth transition from hospital to community is related in no small measure to the CPN who acts as a meaningful bridge-builder between the two settings. The CPN's contact with the resident prior to his final discharge is essential, as is, when applicable, the presence of the resident's relatives at pre-discharge multidisciplinary team meetings.

Day Hospital Attendance

For the person with longer-term mental health problems, the rehabilitation process may need to be continued in a day hospital setting. This applies particularly to those with a diagnosis of schizophrenia who require a degree of help beyond that which was successfully given to Bill by the CPN in the care study described earlier in this chapter.

Attendance at a day hospital not only permits close monitoring, identifying and remedying—if possible—of a client's mental health problems by the multidisciplinary care team, but it also ensures that each attender's care plan is coordinated by his key worker.

Care of the Person in a Long-stay/Sheltered Setting

Today's very much reduced hospital population has, as might be expected, a nucleus of people with high levels of dependency. They have a variety of enduring disabilities and show disturbed behaviours from time to time. It is hoped, nevertheless, that alternative accommodation outside hospital may be possible for most of this group of residents provided daily professional support and supervision is made available.

The aim of care for this resident, regardless of the setting, focuses on improving his quality of life; measures to achieve this include:

- establishing a warm, caring and trusting relationship with a key worker;
- ensuring that problems are not allowed to overshadow strengths and aspirations;
- improving self-esteem by allowing the resident as much control over his daily life as possible;
- empowering him to function at his optimal level of independence.

Identification of Needs and Interventions

To achieve maximum independence. The rehabilitation team will help the resident with the task of becoming as independent of others as is consistent with his mental—and, if elderly, possibly physical—disabilities. Staff support and encouragement is crucial and, as stated above, emphasis is on what the resident *can* do rather than dwelling on his deficits.

The person who has to continue to have at least minimal supervision will also benefit from acquiring or re-establishing many of the everyday practical and social skills outlined above. However, in the early stages the nursing team will need to expend considerable effort in helping the more dependent person initiate new behaviours such as self-care skills. A behavioural approach as advocated by Hall (1983) and Barker and Fraser (1985) often yields positive results. For example, the technique known as chaining is useful to teach a resident to shave himself again after a break of many years. Chaining involves the nurse breaking down a psychomotor skill into manageable units, initially modelling the first step or unit, then physically prompting the individual, if necessary, to try for himself. Successful responses must be immediately reinforced with praise, and encouragement is given to continue. (See Lyttle (1986) for a fuller description of this technique.)

Other equally important outcomes of nursing interventions planned to effect changes in self-care behaviours are the feelings of self-worth and confidence the person experiences as he gradually becomes less and less dependent on others to meet his everyday needs.

To be prevented from becoming institutionalized. The phenomenon of institutionalization was first described by Barton (1959) and Goffman (1961), and is still met with in long-stay wards of psychiatric hospitals (see below). Included in Barton's account is a list of features shown by institutionalized individuals such as apathy, submissiveness and loss of interest in the future. 'Batch living', a term coined by Goffman, describes highly routinized environments within which residents are stripped of their individuality and autonomy and expected to conform to rules imposed by an authoritarian nursing staff. Other classical features of institutionalism are loss of contact with the outside world, few personal possessions, no opportunities for decision-making and a lack of meaningful activities as well as the excessive use of sedating drugs.

One antidote to such impersonal, custodial care is primary nursing. Primary nursing is a patient-centred system of nursing care organization focused on the individual resident's needs rather than the needs of the unit. Each individual resident is allocated a named nurse who is responsible for the planning of that individual resident's care and for the daily monitoring of the quality of his care (see Chapter 4).

In an exploratory study of the nursing care practised in a long-stay psychiatric ward prior to the introduction of primary nursing, Armitage (1988) found institutionalism still in evidence 25 years after the publication of the seminal works cited above. For example, residents, some of whom had an unbroken length in hospital of almost half a century, adhered to a strict routine; there was 'pressure to get patients up and dressed, fed, medicated and bathed before 8.45 a.m.' Staff busied themselves making beds and attending to laundry; little or no time was spent talking with the residents. Any patient–nurse interactions which were observed tended to be exclusively with the more socially competent residents who arguably needed less attention than their more mentally disabled counterparts. Individuals had no choice in the clothes they wore, ward doors were locked due to staff shortages and no arrangements existed for staff and residents to meet together as a group.

Beneficial effects from the introduction of primary nursing included evidence that people were no longer merely passive recipients of nursing care. They had become much more independent of the ward staff and used the opportunities afforded by the weekly community meetings to take part in discussions with the staff on the general running of the ward.

Daily or weekly ward meetings provide an excellent forum for residents in long-term care to make decisions about their living environment and to share information and ideas with the staff. Equally valuable is the potential use of such occasions to help a particular individual to appreciate the effect his actions have on others in the group and to encourage more responsible and accountable patterns of behaviour. Staff behaviours, too, are subject to scrutiny and comment by the more vocal residents; any hint of unilateral decision-making by the staff is identified and justifiably criticized.

In order to prevent the person with long-term mental health problems from becoming institutionalized, the nursing team consistently make every effort to create an environment which is both socially stimulating and psychologically supportive; they also strive to provide as normal and home-like an environment as it is possible to achieve for the residents. Furthermore, the nurse will be available to support an individual resident whenever he is called upon to make his own decisions, and to resist any temptation to intervene should he hesitate. Contact with the outside world is maintained by a plentiful supply of daily newspapers, and discussions of current affairs programmes seen on television take place regularly. Visits to shops and pub lunches provide residents with enjoyable occasions to practise their newly acquired social skills. Holidays at home and abroad, and weekend package tours, all help lay the ghost of institutionalism. At such times residents frquently react favourably to the new responsibilities entrusted to them: accompanying staff report positive responses such as increased sensitivity to the needs of others in the group and of more social interaction generally.

From the residents' perspective, a testimony of the success of a particular trip to London is captured in the words of one who was overheard to say 'It's good to be alive!' (Bentley & Downey, 1989).

Staff Burnout in Long-stay Settings

Positive feedback, such as that from the resident quoted above, is (over)heard less often by psychiatric nurses than by their counterparts in general nursing, and within psychiatric nursing is given more to those working in acute than in long-stay settings. Lack of recognition of one's efforts could lead eventually to low job satisfaction, an early symptom of 'burnout' (McCarthy, 1985). The term burnout was first applied to social workers who showed signs of exhaustion from prolonged exposure to the stress of the caring role. It is defined as: 'A syndrome of physical and emotional exhaustion experienced by those in the helping role when they feel overwhelmed by other people's problems' (Freudenberger, 1974). This phenomenon may progress insidiously, starting with feelings of tiredness from time to time, leading later to regular then chronic feelings of exhaustion with an associated change in attitude towards work. Enthusiasm and high standards of care give way to cynicism; the victim of burnout finally questions the validity of his or her work.

In psychiatric nursing burnout is not confined to any one care setting, but there is some evidence to suggest that the higher the number of patients with schizophrenia in the group the lower is the carer's job satisfaction (Pines & Maslach, 1978). In addition staff working in long-stay facilities may see only limited progress and not infrequent setbacks in the person with longer-term needs, yet they are expected to give him continued and enthusiastic support and encouragement.

Preventing staff burnout requires a measure of informal peer group support and regular supervision and support freely available from concerned and sensitive senior colleagues. Staff development strategies might include formal support groups and opportunities for education in the early recognition of stress-related symptoms. Positive methods of stress reduction should also be included in education programmes.

SUMMARY

This chapter has looked at some of the possible contributing factors to the development of major mental illness, such as schizophrenia, which lead to a break from the real world. It has considered some of the effects that this illness has on the person suffering from it and on the family of the sufferer. It has explored the role of the CPN in caring for people with a schizophrenic condition and shown that the CPN is very much a member of a team of people, both professional colleagues and others working in various voluntary or private organizations. The CPN acts as a coordinator of care and as a provider of care, as a resource person with knowledge of local facilities and as a teacher and educator. The CPN provides support in all the many roles undertaken, but most importantly, the CPN is working with people who suffer from hallucinations and disordered thinking to enable them to live fulfilling and meaningful lives to the best of their abilities out of hospital and in the community. The care of someone requiring to be treated in hospital has been looked at in detail, as have the psychological, physical and social needs that the nurse must consider at all times, both when the person is in an acutely psychotic state and when the person is being prepared for life back in the community. Finally the phenomenon of burnout has been alluded to briefly in the context of staff working in long-stay settings.

FURTHER READING

Brooker C (ed.) (1990) *Community Psychiatric Nursing: A Research Perspective*. London: Chapman & Hall.

Brooker C & White E (1993) *Community Psychiatric Nursing: A Research Perspective*, volume 2. London: Chapman & Hall.

Brooking J, Ritter S & Thomas B (eds) (1992) *A Textbook of Psychiatric and Mental Health Nursing*. Edinburgh: Churchill Livingstone.

Community Psychiatric Nursing Association Journals.

Cronin-Stubbs D & Brophy E (1985) Burnout: can social support save the psychiatric nurse? *Journal of Psychosocial Nursing* **23**(7): 8–13.

Hume C & Pullen I (1994) *Rehabilitation for Mental Health Problems*. Edinburgh: Churchill Livingstone.

Mertzankis L (1990) Improving social skills. *Nursing Times* **86**(44): 44–46.

Simmons S & Brooker C (1986) *Community Psychiatric Nursing: A Social Perspective*. London: Heinemann.

Warner C (1989) Actions speak louder than words. *Nursing Times* **85**(22): 70–71.

REFERENCES

Affleck J & McGuire R (1984) The measurement of psychiatric rehabilitation status. A review of the needs and a new scale. *British Journal of Psychiatry* **145**: 517–525.

Armitage P (1988) Changing care: an evaluation of primary nursing in psychiatric long term care. School of Nursing Studies, University of Wales College of Medicine, Cardiff.

Atkinson J (1986) *Schizophrenia at Home: A Guide to Helping the Family*. London: Croom Helm.

Barker P (1985) *Patient Assessment in Psychiatric Nursing*. London: Croom Helm.

Barker P & Fraser D (1985) Rehabilitation in psychiatric and mentally handicapped hospitals. In: Barker P & Fraser D (eds) *The Nurse as a Therapist: A Behavioural Approach*. London: Croom Helm.

Barton R (1959) *Institutional Neurosis*. Bristol: Wright.

Bentley J & Downey M (1989) Advance to Mayfair. *Nursing Times* **85**(29): 57–59.

Cutting J (1989) Hearing voices. *British Medical Journal* **289**: 769–770.

Farr E (1982) A personal account of schizophrenia. In: Tsuang M (ed.) *Schizophrenia: The Facts*. Oxford: Oxford University Press.

Freudenberger H (1974) Staff burnout. *Journal of Social Issues* **30**(i): 159–166.

Goffman E (1961) *Asylums*. Harmondsworth: Penguin.

Goldberg D & Huxley P (1980) *Mental Illness in the Community: The Pathway to Psychiatric Care*. London: Tavistock.

Hall J (1983) Ward based rehabilitation programmes. In: Watts F & Bennett D (eds) *Theory and Practice of Psychiatric Rehabilitation*. Chichester: Wiley.

Heston L (1966) Psychiatric disorders in foster home reared children of schizophrenic mothers. *British Journal of Psychiatry* **112**: 819–825.

Hiles P (1984) Schizophrenia: an inside story. *New Society* **68**(1125): 439–440.

HMSO (1989) *Caring for People. Community Care in the Next Decade and Beyond: Policy Guidance*. London: HMSO.

Jenkins R, Field V & Young R (1992) *The Primary Care of Schizophrenia*. London: HMSO.

Kringlen E (1987) Contributions of genetic studies on schizophrenia. In: Hafner H, Gattaz W, Janzarik (eds) *Search for the Causes of Schizophrenia*. Berlin: Springer-Verlag.

Leff L & Vaughn C (1985) *Expressed Emotion in Families: Its Significance for Mental Illness*. New York: Guildford Press.

Lyttle J (1986) *Mental Disorder: Its Care and Treatment*. London: Baillière Tindall, pp. 127–128.

McCarthy P (1985) Burnout in psychiatric nursing. *Journal of Advanced Nursing* **10**: 305–310.

Macauley R (1989) Back to school. *Nursing Times* **83**(3): 35–37.

Margo A, Hemsley D & Slade P (1981) The effects of varying auditory input on schizophrenic hallucinations. *British Journal of Psychiatry* **139**: 122–127.

National Schizophrenia Fellowship (1974) *Social Provision for Sufferers from Chronic Schizophrenia*. Surbiton: NSF.

National Schizophrenia Fellowship (1975) *Schizophrenia—The Family Burden*. Surbiton: NSF.

Pines A & Maslach C (1978) Characteristics of staff burnout in Mental Health settings. *Hospital and Community Psychiatry* **89**(4): 233–237.

Robinson A (1984) Rock and roll delusions. *British Journal of Psychiatry* **145**: 672.

Sartorius N, Jablensky A, Korten A *et al.* (1986) Early manifestations and first-contact incidence of schizophrenia in different cultures. *Psychological Medicine* **16**: 909–928.

Shelton R & Weinberger D (1986) X-ray computerised tomography studies in schizophrenia: a review and synthesis. In: Nasrallah H & Weinberger D (eds) *The Neurology of Schizophrenia*. Amsterdam: Elsevier.

Trower P, Bryant B & Argyle M (1978) *Social Skills and Mental Health*. London: Methuen.

Warner R (1985) *Recovery from Schizophrenia*. London: Routledge & Kegan Paul.

World Health Organization (1979) *Schizophrenia: An International Follow-up Study*. Chichester: John Wiley & Sons.

Chapter 10
Caring for the Elderly Person who is Confused

INTRODUCTION

This chapter will consider first of all *acute confusion* in the elderly person who is being cared for in the hospital setting. Confusion may also be *chronic*, and is frequently given the term 'dementia'. Care of the person with dementia will then be described, firstly in the community, followed by care of this person when needs change and care has to be continued in a hospital setting.

The psychological needs of the chronically confused elderly person in hospital will be emphasized in this chapter. Details of the care required to meet this elderly person's physical needs, such as the nursing measures to help promote urinary continence, are fully covered in texts specifically devoted to the care of elderly people (see Further Reading).

Acute Confusion

Causes of acute confusion in the elderly are numerous and include:

- infections, particularly chest and urinary infections;
- vascular disorders, for example cerebrovascular accidents, subdural haematoma due to falls;
- anoxia, as associated with biventricular failure;
- electrolyte imbalance;

- polypharmacy, i.e. the prescribing of too many drugs for too many conditions;
- hypo- and hyperglycaemia;
- hypothermia.

Once the underlying cause of the acute confusion has been found and treated, complete recovery can be expected in the majority of patients.

The most prominent symptoms are clouding of consciousness, disorientation for time and place, and disturbance of memory for recent events. The patient is unable to understand what is happening around him. His attention wanders; he misidentifies people and often fails to recognize familiar objects. His actions may appear strange because he may carry out correct movements but in the wrong circumstances; for example, he may try to write with a cigarette, or eat soap, because he is unable to identify the object he is using. He may have hallucinatory experiences; he may see terrifying visions, or behave as if he were responding to voices. Following some infections, the cardinal symptoms are tiredness, irritability and depression. Whenever the picture is one of acute confusion it is important, by means of careful examination, to establish a diagnosis of the physical disorder and institute appropriate treatment.

Effects of Different Types of Dementia

As already stated the term 'dementia' is frequently given to the condition of chronic confusion and will be used interchangeably throughout the rest of the chapter.

The word dementia has come to be applied very loosely to all those people above a certain age who present with a degree of memory loss, altered behaviour patterns and a general deterioration in their awareness of time, place and person. It should only be used when referring either to specific diseases, such as presenile or senile dementia, or to a disease syndrome which indicates 'an acquired global impairment of intellect, memory and personality' leading to a chronic, widespread dysfunction of the brain (Lishman, 1987).

Research continues to try to disentangle the exact causes of the ageing process, to establish what contributes to one person becoming old gracefully while another person becomes confused, disorientated, forgetful and seems to become a totally different person from the one the family members knew and loved and respected.

The presenile dementias, which include those diseases which begin to show signs and symptoms before the age of 65 years, for example Pick's disease, Huntington's chorea and Creutzfeldt–Jakob's disease, appear to show a predisposition for a genetic origin, with a single dominant gene having been identified in many cases of Huntington's chorea. Modern techniques of molecular biology now make it possible to predict, in a proportion of cases, which individuals at risk are destined to develop the disease. There is growing evidence that there are other neurochemical and neurobiological factors which may be susceptible to prevention and treatment and this gives rise to hopes that these conditions may be helped in the future.

One of the most common types of chronic organic psychiatric disorder (see p. 303) is 'senile dementia' also referred to as senile dementia of the Alzheimer type (SDAT) because post-mortem changes in senile dementia are virtually identical with those occurring in Alzheimer's disease (a form of presenile dementia). The cause is as yet unknown, though, according to some researchers in this field, findings suggestive of brain-enzyme abnormalities have yielded some encouraging results. One in five persons over 80 years of age is affected. Women are more likely to develop this disorder than men. These changes in the brain include neurofibrillary tangles and senile plaques in the cortex of the brain which are common in all people as they grow older. However, these changes appear to be four times greater in those who subsequently require admission to hospital because their condition becomes too severe to be cared for in the community.

Another type of dementia is known as *atherosclerotic* or *multi-infarct dementia*. The smaller blood vessels in the brain become blocked due to atherosclerosis, or the accumulation of fatty deposits on the inside walls of the blood vessels. This reduces the flow of oxygen and nutrients to the brain and the elimination of toxic substances from the brain, which leads to the destruction of the normal functioning of the brain. There may well be a combination of these two types of dementia which causes the state of chronic confusion to develop.

The onset of dementia is usually seen when people reach 70 to 80 years of life and is more common in females than in males. It is usually very insidious, often being put down to the normal processes of ageing, and only becomes an issue following a particular emergency or acute episode of change or illness. It usually manifests itself in changes in memory, in behaviour patterns and in personality:

- memory begins to fail;
- people become inefficient, muddled over ordinary everyday tasks;
- they lose interest and initiative in past hobbies and activities;

- they may become perplexed, agitated and restless, partly due to the growing inability to make sense of the world around them.

Elderly people may begin to show an exaggeration of character traits such as obstinancy, and rigidity to old habits. There may be problems:

- with transferring thoughts into coherent speech;
- with performing some voluntary movements;
- with recognition of family members.

With SDAT there is usually a blunting of the emotions and a lack of insight into the progression of the condition, unlike the multi-infarct cause of dementia when there is considerable fluctuation in the course of the disease, with periods of clarity and lucidity when awareness can lead to more anxiety and depression. It is therefore important for the nurse who is caring for a number of people with dementia to be very aware of each individual's mental state and needs.

MEETING THE NEEDS OF THE ACUTELY CONFUSED ELDERLY PERSON IN HOSPITAL

A primary need of the acutely confused elderly person is to be looked after in a safe physical and psychological environment, to be *closely observed* for unpredictable behaviour such as trying to 'escape' from frightening visual or tactile hallucinations. The elderly person may try to climb out of a window or rush along the corridor and out of the main door. Ideally, the acutely confused person ought to be nursed in a single room, cared for by only three or four nurses in total, as occurs in units where primary nursing is practised, rather than being confronted by a succession of unfamiliar faces throughout the day and night. The presence of a relative or close friend can reduce the restlessness of the elderly person, especially at night.

The use of non-verbal communication, a hand gently held or stroked and an affectionate hug are very reassuring for the confused elderly person who is bewildered, perplexed and often extremely agitated by his inability to understand what is happening to him.

It helps the elderly person when explanations are kept simple and are clearly spoken. Concentration is very poor and attention span is of short duration, necessitating frequent repetition of information.

Disorientation for time and place is lessened by large clocks and calendars, hospital booklets and charts, and verbal reminders from the nursing team of the name of the hospital and the ward or unit. The use of spectacles and a hearing aid, if normally worn, prevents sensory deprivation—another factor to be considered when helping the confused elderly person in his struggle to make sense of his surroundings.

In a condition where the patient is experiencing fluctuating levels of consciousness, lucid periods may be utilized to help meet his nutritional needs and reality is reinforced whenever possible by allowing him to drink or eat a light diet without assistance.

An elderly person suffering from an acute confusional state is often physically very ill and nursing interventions will include regular recording of the patient's vital signs, assisting him to meet personal and oral hygiene and elimination needs, and maintaining the integrity of his skin.

MEETING THE NEEDS OF THE PERSON WITH CHRONIC CONFUSION IN THE COMMUNITY

In looking at the physical, psychological and social needs of the person with dementia the progress of a hypothetical patient will be followed; the various phases of the disease and the needs of both the sufferer and the family in coping at the different stages will be considered, and the different agencies and organizations identified that may be available to help make life tolerable and to enable the person to remain in her chosen, familiar environment for as long as possible with a reasonable quality of life.

CARE STUDY

Mrs Mary Lees lives in a three bedroomed house with her husband in the street to which they came as a young married couple 45 years ago.

She is 69 years old and her husband, Jim, is 73.

They have three children who are all married: one daughter lives in Canada, another in London and the third child, a son, lives in the same town, twenty minute's drive away.

Mrs Lees has always been an active member of the local community; for years she ran the cub group; she was a keen member of the Womens' Institute and the Mothers' Union. Sadly, her husband's increasing physical ill-health has caused her to reduce some of her activities so that she can be at home to help nurse him. However, recently, Mrs Lees has begun to show subtle changes in her own behaviour. For example, she has mixed up and forgotten to give her husband his correct medication; she has been a little erratic in the household shopping, buying items that she did not need and forgetting essentials such as tea and butter. On one occasion she arrived at a meeting that she had not attended for many months, causing some consternation when she tried to take over some duties she had carried out in times past. Her daughter, Mrs Muriel Grant, visiting from London, began to feel some concern about what was happening to her mother and talked things over with her brother and sister-in-law who, though they had been visiting regularly, said they had not noticed anything particularly alarming. (This illustrates the difference in perception between those who are close to a situation and who may not notice gradual deterioration in social functioning and those who may perceive greater change from less frequent contact).

Mrs Grant decided to contact her mother's GP partly to enquire about the general well-being of both her parents, and partly to make known her own anxiety about her mother's ability to cope with everything. The GP promised to look into things on his next visit to her father. Following his visit to Mr and Mrs Lees at their home he referred Mrs Lees to the local consultant psychogeriatrician who, in this instance, made a domiciliary visit with the community psychiatric nurse for the elderly. Together they made an initial assessment of Mrs Lees's physical and mental state, of her social situation and need for support. Over a period of time the team for the care of the elderly met with those members of the family who were available and discussed what would be a reasonable plan of care for the two elderly people, each with their different needs. It was agreed that the CPN would be the care coordinator for the family, to whom they could turn for information and support at each change in the condition or circumstances of their parents.

As Mr Lees's physical condition deteriorated and Mrs Lees could no longer cope, he had to be admitted to a nursing home, in spite of the interventions of both the district nurse and the community care assistant who had been going in to help Mrs Lees with the daily tasks of running a home and caring for a sick partner. Mrs Lees beame very distressed by her husband's admission and showed greater signs of muddle and disorientation. Following a review of her situation it became necessary for her, too, to be admitted into hospital for a period of assessment, during which time her physical health was thoroughly investigated to eliminate or identify any underlying physical condition.

The team social worker met with members of the family to negotiate how much help and support they would be able to offer Mrs Lees on her return home. They discussed whether it would be better for Mrs Lees to stay in her own home or move into some kind of sheltered accommodation such as a warden controlled flat. Neither Mrs Lees nor the family wanted her to have to move out of her home so they agreed to a plan that would enable them to share the burden of care, with help and support from the CPN.

Care Programme for Mrs Lees

1   Mrs Lees would attend the day centre run by Age Concern two days a week.
2   A volunteer driver would take her each week to visit her husband in his nursing home as worry about him had largely contributed to her mental deterioration.
3   Mr and Mrs Lees (Junior) would call in daily to make sure she had all that she required and that she was managing to cope.
4   Mrs Grant would come from London to stay once a fortnight at the weekends to relieve her brother and his wife.
5   The family was put in touch with their respective branches of the Alzheimer's Disease Society who were able to give invaluable advice and support through their local groups.
6   A regular review of Mrs Lees's care would be made, with

the CPN as coordinator calling a meeting of all those involved in her care.

7   Respite care would be agreed, if the family decided that present arrangements required changing. This might entail Mrs Lees going into hospital for a short period at regular intervals in order to help the family to cope more easily.

The overall aims of this care programme are to enable Mrs Lees to maintain as much independence as possible and to allow her to live in her own home for as long as possible, to maximize the abilities she retains and to help her in those areas that have become more difficult. It has to be acknowledged, however, that Mrs Lees may deteriorate and require admission to hospital.

CARING FOR THE ELDERLY PERSON WITH CHRONIC CONFUSION IN HOSPITAL

Sadly, but not unexpectedly, Mrs Lees's dementia did deteriorate and she was admitted to a unit for the elderly mentally ill within her local psychiatric hospital.

Many of Mrs Lees's present needs are not dissimilar to those described while she was still at home but as Mrs Lees's dementia advances so the nurse has to become more and more resourceful in her efforts to maintain meaningful communication patterns with her. The nursing team who care for people like Mrs Lees face a considerable challenge as they try to help their patients experience a lessening of their sense of isolation—due partly to communication difficulties—and an increase in feelings of self-worth.

The following are possible therapeutic strategies

which may be tried to meet the psychological needs of Mrs Lees and others who suffer from this progressive and tragic condition.

Reality Orientation

Reality orientation (RO) is the term applied to a number of therapeutic approaches designed to promote the chronically confused elderly person's contact with reality. In addition to the steps taken to lessen the disorientation for time, place and person associated with the acutely confused elderly person, described earlier in this chapter, modifications to the environment include:

- a large 'orientation board' placed in a prominent position stating day (changed daily!) date and weather in large clearly visible lettering;
- clear signs or symbols indicating significant areas such as the kitchen, bedrooms and toilets;
- a line of carpet tiles of a distinctive colour indicating the way to toilets.

Holden and Woods (1982) describe two specific techniques.

Informal (or 24 Hour) Reality Orientation

Using this technique the carer takes advantage of all interactions with the person to reinforce reality. On approach the confused person is greeted by his or her preferred name and the carer reintroduces herself, refers to the time of day and perhaps the weather. Touch is useful to focus the person's attention and gain eye contact. Clear brief sentences are used to explain what is about to be done, and information is repeated as necessary. Incorrect responses are gently corrected.

Thus a night nurse, seeing a disoriented elderly person wandering around in the early hours might, say:

'Hello, Mr Scott, I'm Mary Green, the night nurse. It's two o'clock in the morning . . .' rather than 'Mr Scott why are you not in bed at this time? Where are you going? What is the matter?'

Class (or Formal) Reality Orientation

This involves small group sessions and is suitable for people who, though not severely organically impaired, are nevertheless apathetic and socially withdrawn. Two or three times a week, or sometimes daily, the same group of people meet for approximately half an hour at the same time of day. A therapist, who may be a nurse or another member of the multidisciplinary care team, talks with the elderly people about a variety of different topics such as the weather, food, holidays or past personal events. In essence, the aim is to reinstate existing memories rather than to attempt to create new ones.

It may be, however, that by the time Mrs Lees has to be admitted to hospital on a long-term basis, the severity of her intellectual functioning is such that the approaches used in reality orientation are of little or no benefit to her. One or more of the following therapeutic options may be of more value.

Reminiscence Therapy

As the name suggests, the importance of this therapy rests largely on its being able to capitalize on one of the patient's few remaining assets in terms of cognitive functioning, a relatively intact long-term memory with its retrievable store of past experiences. A number of people with varying degrees of intellectual impairment respond positively to reminiscence stimulus materials, for example old photographs of local interest and wartime memorabilia. Using a four-point scale to indicate areas of verbal and non-verbal communication such as initiating interaction, responding and facial expression, Griffiths and Burford (1988) found some improvement had taken place in the competencies of the members of their weekly group. This therapeutic tool can remind the elderly person, and also inform his listeners, of his former achievements and of the noteworthy contributions to life he has made in the past. As with reality orientation, reminiscence therapy can be practised successfully on an informal basis. The nurse sets time aside throughout the day to give her undivided attention to the patient, who is encouraged to use the opportunity to relive positive experiences from his past. Such occasions can be of special benefit to the elderly person, who, in his present circumstances, has a dwindling number of new and interesting experiences, as his physical health as well as mental health follow a progressively downhill course.

Validation Therapy

When caring for the person whose intellectual impairment is very severe, it may be that a nurse's repeated attempts to orientate him to the present, using reality orientation techniques, are of doubtful relevance, and may serve only to increase his distress and sense of isolation. It was dissatisfaction with such reality orientation measures which led Feil (1982) to develop an alternative approach to care, known as validation therapy. One of the basic assumptions of this therapy is that although the severely disoriented person's speech may make little or no sense to the listener it does have meaning for the speaker. The nurse should listen carefully to the words and respond appropriately to the underlying feeling tone in an effort to convey empathy and ease the person's distress.

Sometimes, the repetition of a word or phrase by the nurse may assist the person to express himself further. For example, when the patient says 'I want to go home', the nurse might reply, 'What do you miss most about home?' or 'What would you like to do at home?' The appropriate use of reminiscing—an integral part of validation therapy—may also be encouraged by the nurse and can often prove to be a pleasurable experience for this patient.

Comparing reality orientation with validation therapy, Morton and Bleathman (1988) state that by 'using validation, we talk to the disoriented on *their* ground, on *their* terms, on the subjects *they* raise and choose to discuss'. Feil (1982) goes further and asserts that validation therapy facilitates the demented person to resolve past conflicts, the existence of which have, until the present, been repressed or denied by him.

Touch—a Therapeutic Tool

Touch is essential for the well-being of all individuals at every stage of life, in illness or in health, and in the care of a severely demented person it can be one of the most effective ways of establishing personal contact. Its use can convey concern and give comfort when words have lost some of their meaning. A warm hug from the nurse, or an affectionate squeeze of the elderly person's hand can help ease distress and lessen feelings of isolation.

The use of basic hand massage can also decrease feelings of isolation and can lift communication barriers between patient and nurse. Gentle stroking movements applied to the hands, and, for some people to the feet, can gradually induce a relaxed response in an agitated elderly person. In addition to massage, Wise (1989) recommends the use of the aroma of certain essential oils—a few drops added to a bowl of hot water placed nearby—to promote relaxation and a sense of well-being.

Music Therapy

For those whose minds have lost so much, song and rhyme may still be an invaluable medium for communication. In addition to formal music therapy sessions, opportunities taken to sing favourite hymns and songs popular in patients' younger years, or to recite well-loved verse, may produce surprisingly rewarding results. In an evocative line, Brooker (1991) observes that 'seemingly "lost" elderly confused patients . . . "come alive" in response to a singalong session'.

RELATIVE SUPPORT GROUPS

Following admission of an elderly relative into hospital, feelings of guilt and distress are often exacerbated within the carers and family members. Relative Support Groups can be particularly helpful in allowing people to give voice to their feelings, in sharing problems and difficulties, in giving advice and support to one another so that caring members of families do not feel so alone with their thoughts and problems. These groups are held both in the community for those who are caring for elderly people in their homes and in hospital for those whose elderly relatives need to be cared for in a hospital setting.

Whatever care programme may be agreed, whether in the community or in hospital, it is always essential to involve the carers and family members. They provide by far the greatest amount of care for elderly people who remain at home and will continue to do so. They may be willing to care but they may also have their own worries associated with their own families, with their work and their own lives, which make it difficult to do as much as they might like. They may feel guilty and distressed at their own inability to cope, or their own reluctance to take on a caring role due to any number of circumstances. They themselves will need much sensitive support to manage their own ambivalent and confused feelings. The Relative Support Group can contribute to this support. The CPN is a key person who can get to know the family well and offer advice or support as and when it is needed.

Not enough attention has been given in the past to the needs of those caring for confused, elderly people at home. There have been too many assumptions made that carers know all about the cause, onset and prognosis of dementia; that they are informed about the different services and benefits that they may claim; that they know how to contact the various services and agencies concerned with the elderly. A collaborative approach to care is becoming the norm, in which doctors, nurses, social workers, occupational therapists, psychologists all recognize that for a programme of care to be successful, it is essential to include the patient, and the person most directly involved in the daily caring, in all discussions.

They all need to know and understand the practical problems that have to be faced every day and together decide on realistic ways of overcoming them. The CPN, by working closely with other colleagues, can coordinate care, monitor that it happens, and evaluate how effective and successful it is. Relative Support Groups to which carers can bring their worries and experiences can provide an opportunity for CPNs to pick up where gaps in service exist or where information and practical solutions are missing. An alert CPN can quickly pick up clues when stress and anxiety are developing, and can take active measures to alleviate unnecessary distress.

It is important to remember that elderly people are no different to others in wishing to preserve their dignity as individuals. They may begin to need help with the daily activities of living, they may be confused at times, forgetful, muddled, but, if they thought at all of the consequences of growing old they must have hoped that they would always be treated and considered with respect for the person that they are and have been. Nurses need to work together with carers to enable them to continue wanting to care and to care effectively, feeling supported in their own right so that looking after confused, elderly people in their own homes is much less of a burden but becomes a pleasure with a sense of fulfilment.

When an elderly person requires to be cared for in hospital the need to work with carers continues and nurses must be sensitive to allowing and encouraging relatives to continue doing what they can, such as helping to feed them, taking them for walks or outings in the grounds of the hospital, looking after their laundry if they so wish, so that relatives still have a sense of involvement, which can help to lessen the feelings of guilt and abandonment that relatives sometimes feel when they are no longer able to care for their loved ones at home.

SUMMARY

In this chapter the different needs of the acutely confused elderly person and the elderly person with chronic confusion, or dementia, have been discussed. Emphasis has been placed on caring for people in their own homes for as long as possible, if this is what both the elderly person and the family wish. Nurses, as members of a wider team, have an important role in coordinating care and providing support to the families, whether the elderly person is living in the community or requires to be nursed in hospital. For many, the provision of respite care enables relatives to continue caring at home, and nurses can provide the continuity in each setting. Wherever care takes place, elderly people deserve to be treated with respect and dignity, in a safe and caring environment.

FURTHER READING

Brooker C (ed.) (1990) *Community Psychiatric Nursing—A Research Perspective*. London: Chapman & Hall.

Brooker C & White E (eds) (1993) *Community Psychiatric Nursing—A Research Perspective*, Volume 2. London: Chapman & Hall.

McCann K (1991) Elderly patients' perception of touch. *Nursing Times* **87**(16): 53.

Watson R (1993) *Caring for Elderly People*. London: Baillière Tindall.

REFERENCES

Brooker E (1991) Just a song at twilight. *Nursing Times* **87**(38): 32–34.

Feil N (1982) *Validation—The Feil Method*. Cleveland: Edward Feil Productions.

Griffiths H & Burford A (1988) Thanks for the memory. *Nursing Times* **84**(36): 55–56.

Holden V & Woods R (1982) *Reality Orientation*. Edinburgh: Churchill Livingstone.

Lishman WA (1987) *Organic Psychiatry. The Psychological Consequences of Cerebral Disorder*. Oxford: Blackwell Scientific Publications.

Morton I & Bleathman C (1988) Reality orientation: Does it matter whether it's Tuesday or Friday? *Nursing Times* **84**(6): 25–27.

Wise R (1989) Flower Power. *Nursing Times* **85**(22): 45–47.

Chapter 11
Caring for the Person who is Anxious

INTRODUCTION

Anxiety is something we all experience. In some instances it is necessary for survival as it stimulates us to take the actions needed to escape dangerous situations. This chapter looks at what constitutes normal anxiety, identifies the signs and symptoms of anxiety, considers some of the causes of anxiety, and finally, explores how psychiatric nurses can meet the needs of the anxious person.

NORMAL ANXIETY

Anxiety is an emotion that is a part of everyday life. Most people learn to live with it and accept it without having to say consciously 'I feel anxious because . . .' every time they face an uncomfortable situation. They have learned to be alert to potential danger and to take action to avoid or minimize the danger. For example, whenever one wishes to cross the road one knows that one must check that there is no traffic coming, that it is safe to cross over to the other side, or that, although a car is coming it is far enough away to cross if one walks swiftly. There may be an element of risk but one can cope with that risk without feeling that something catastrophic will happen. One may become aware that the heart is thumping a little more, breath is coming faster as one steps out quickly, that one feels hotter and more stimulated when the other side of the road is reached, but these sensations are not troublesome; they are accepted and taken for granted. Most people have experienced pre-exam nerves, the anxiety associated with meeting new people, or having a first driving lesson. Thoughts such as 'Will I make a fool of myself?' or 'What will happen if I fail?' or 'What if he doesn't like me?' go through the mind and certain physiological responses become noticeable. These may be unpleasant while they last, but it is known that they will pass without any disaster occurring. In fact, the physiological responses to anxiety can in many instances assist people to behave and perform better than if they were entirely laid back and indifferent to the outcome of their actions.

It may be helpful to try to distinguish between *anxiety* and *fear*. Marks (1978) in his book *'Living With Fear – Understanding and Coping with Anxiety'* says that 'the feeling of anxiety is closely related to that of fear and similar emotions . . . when the cause of the worry is readily apparent, we tend to call the emotion *fear'*. He uses the example of the emotion experienced when facing a charging lion. The cause of the emotional response is very clear. However, when the emotion felt is of a less disturbing nature, giving rise to feelings of unease and discomfort, it is described as *anxiety*. Only when the feelings become so great that they lead to the avoidance of normal activity and affect the way people can live their lives and make relationships, do the feelings of fear and anxiety become problematic. At present, we do not know exactly why different people cope with similar situations in different ways. Some people appear able to cope with much greater levels of stress than others. This may in part be due to genetic make-up and may in part be influenced by environment and upbringing. There has been much research into the way children learn certain behaviours, how early experiences affect the way we behave in adulthood and how that learned behaviour can be handed down from parent to child, thus perpetuating possible poor ways of coping with difficulties faced throughout life.

PHYSIOLOGICAL SIGNS OF ANXIETY

The body's defence mechanisms are programmed in such a way as to assist people to react when threatened. The autonomic nervous system automatically goes into action when it receives certain messages. This has been called the 'fight or flight' response. If the body perceives a dangerous situation it prepares itself to deal with the situation.

- The heart begins to pump more strongly and rapidly in order to provide the muscles with more blood in preparation for an increase in activity.
- Pulse rate becomes faster.
- Breathing becomes shallower and more rapid to increase the amount of oxygen circulating in the bloodstream.
- Perspiration appears on the surface of the body to cool it after exertion.
- Muscles contract as tension increases.
- Sphincters constrict leading to feelings of nausea or a desire to urinate.

It is as though the body is shutting down on all unnecessary activities and preparing for action.

Other subjective descriptions of changes in the body due to the autonomic nervous system include:

- dryness of the mouth;
- shakiness in the hands and legs or 'legs like jelly';
- sweaty palms;
- 'butterflies in the stomach';
- feelings of unreality;
- a desire to cry;
- feelings of light-headedness and as though about to fall or faint.

The body is preparing either to flee from the danger or to become still and face the danger. All of these symptoms are normal reactions to the dangers we face day by day.

PSYCHOLOGICAL REACTIONS TO FEAR

These are the *thoughts* that accompany the consciousness of experiencing the physiological symptoms, so that the way a person perceives and interprets what is happening can influence the way he or she reacts to events in the future. Very young children experience anxiety when they are separated from their parents whom they have learned to depend on to fulfil their basic needs such as food, warmth, comfort and security. They cry when mother or father does not appear, and brighten up considerably when they return. Usually, parents do reappear, and the child learns to accept a certain amount of anxiety. When a child does not have a stable figure on whom to depend but is constantly left with feelings of doubt and insecurity it grows up with less of an ability to trust others. The child may grow up fiercely independent, having learned at a very early age that in order to survive he has to fight for his share, or the child grows up anxious, unable to achieve his potential, always fearful, unable to make satisfactory relationships, partly because he is wanting others to look after him and make decisions for him. He doubts his ability to make sensible judgements or to distinguish between fact and fantasy, real and imagined dangers.

In normal development people learn through their experiences and interactions with other people what they are likely to feel and how they should behave in given circumstances. They are usually able to find acceptable reasons for why certain things happen. They may not like the outcome of their behaviour or the effect someone else's behaviour has on them, but they are able to use their reasoning powers to explain the consequences of particular actions.

Thoughts such as 'I feel anxious' or 'I feel frightened' may be quite reasonable in given situations:

'I feel anxious that I may fail this exam because I have not done enough revision' is a perfectly appropriate response.

'I feel anxious that I may fail this exam even though I have worked hard all year and spent hours revising the work of the year' may appear an inappropriate response with a disproportionate expectation of failure.

'I am afraid to walk down that street now as there is a riot going on and I may be hurt' is a reasonable appraisal of present conditions.

'I am afraid of ever going down that street because the last time I came this way there was a riot going on' would seem to be an exaggerated response, overgeneralizing a previous experience. Somehow the fear experienced and the thoughts that accompanied that fear have become distorted.

Research with patients who have presented with problems of anxiety and abnormal fears has demonstrated that these emotions have arisen from faulty interpretations and perceptions of events, when not enough information was available which led to mistakes in distinguishing between reality and imagination (Beck, 1976).

The ability to cope with the problems that life brings depends greatly on how people regard themselves and on their attitude to themselves and to others. If one's thinking is directed by feelings of good self-image, high self-esteem, a strong sense of identity, a fair degree or optimism and hope, then it is highly likely that one will be able to deal with the knocks that come one's way. If, on the other hand, one has a poor self-image, with a low self-esteem and a confused sense of identity, it is more likely that one will have a distorted outlook on life and faulty expectations of what life may bring.

TYPES OF ANXIETY AND FEAR

Although anxiety is a normal part of life there are situations when anxiety becomes disabling and interferes with an individual's ability to perform everyday tasks that most people take for granted. The feelings that arise can be expressed on a continuum from mild general anxiety to full-blown paralysing panic attacks at the mere thought of facing a particular situation or specific object.

Anxiety States

The basis of anxiety is 'worry' which over a period of time becomes persistent and excessive. It can occur 'out of the blue', with no recognizable trigger. A general title of 'free floating anxiety' used to be given to this type of anxiety. People experience a number of physical symptoms which suddenly descend on them or sweep over them at any time of the day or night. The feelings are usually transitory, and disappear after a few minutes, but can last for some hours. Sometimes they may occur only once or twice a day. With some people they can reoccur at more frequent intervals and although they pass, the sufferer remains feeling drained and tremulous between episodes. In some instances, the condition can be so debilitating that the person concerned is forced to leave work and remain at home. A vicious circle develops whereby a person feels so anxious that he stops going out and becomes preoccupied with the physical symptoms and is convinced that he is suffering from an incurable disease or is about to have a heart attack.

Phobic Disorders or Phobias

A phobic anxiety state can be triggered by virtually any object or situation. We are all familiar with people who are particularly frightened of spiders, or cats or dogs. Many people suffer from a fear of heights or of being in enclosed spaces. The most common syndrome amongst the phobic anxiety states is that described as *agoraphobia*, and many people suffering from depression also describe agoraphobic symptoms. These include:

- fear of being in the open;
- fear of being in shops and especially of having to queue at check-outs;
- fear of being among crowds, whether in the street or at a football match;
- fear of being in enclosed spaces such as a lift, bus, train, theatre or cinema;
- fear of any form of travel, e.g. aeroplanes, ships, as well as the above;

- fear of crossing bridges;
- fear of being alone at home.

It appears to occur more often in women, starting in young adulthood, but does not appear to have any particular pattern of precipitating factors. Many people are able to disguise the degree of fear that they are suffering by adopting various strategies for helping them to cope, such as having something to hold on to, an umbrella, a shopping trolley, a push-bike. If they do manage to go out to the cinema or to church they will insist on sitting in an aisle seat so that they can go out quickly when the feelings of panic become too intense. Some of the other more common areas of phobia are listed below:

- social phobias
- illness phobias
- animal phobias
- noise phobia

Obsessive–Compulsive States/Disorders

These disorders, when they occur, frequently include an obsessive thought which can only be alleviated by compulsive rituals. The thoughts keep coming into the mind, time and time again, even against the will, and often carry with them the fear of some impending disaster. This disaster will only be avoided if the person performs certain tasks which take on the function of a ritual. People suffering from obsessive–compulsive disorders usually know that what they are thinking and doing is irrational but they are powerless to prevent themselves from completing the ritual due to the force of the fear driving them. Fear of contamination or fear of causing harm to others or of being harmed oneself are the most frequent causes of obsessive–compulsive disorders. These fears lead sufferers to perform complicated rituals that usually consist of time-consuming hand-washing, bathing or house-cleaning. These rituals can so interfere with the sufferers' life that they are unable to go to work, or enjoy a walk down the street. Family members can be drawn into the ritual process and relationships with both family and friends can be badly disrupted.

TREATMENT FOR ANXIETY, PHOBIAS AND OBSESSIVE–COMPULSIVE DISORDERS

The overriding objective behind all treatment programmes for these conditions is to enable sufferers to take control of their own feelings. As a certain amount of anxiety and fear is healthy, natural and to be welcomed in certain situations, it should not be the aim of the therapist to remove all fear and anxiety, but to help the person to face the difficult situations without being so crippled or disabled by the feelings that accompany the thoughts or actions. This is achieved through learning not to avoid the fearful situation, but to face the fear. 'There is nothing so fearful as the fear of the fear itself.'

The quickest and most successful method of achieving this, is, according to Marks (1978), through exposure to the feared situation. This may take time and require much effort, patience and determination, but the results are very rewarding and lasting. Research and experience in the clinical field has shown that whatever the degree of anxiety or panic a person feels at the thought of doing something, or even actually doing it, sooner or later that level of anxiety subsides and the person is none the worse for it. Careful preparation, thorough explanation of everything that may happen, clear and firm instructions, given in a sensitive and encouraging manner that engenders a willingness to continue in therapy, will all contribute to a successful outcome. Treatment may take the form of:

- *systematic desensitization*—gradual exposure from the least frightening to progressively more difficult situations;
- *flooding*—exposure in imagination through 'fantasy', using films, slides, pictures, etc.; to exposure in real life to the worst possible anxiety-provoking situations;
- *paradoxical intention*—instructing the person to achieve the very thing he is afraid of;
- *cognitive techniques*—challenging automatic negative thoughts, negative self-statements, distorted beliefs about the consequences of actions; use of 'cue cards' as reminders; distraction.

Treatment programmes may be carried out with the individual alone or in groups with other sufferers when group members are able to give each other encouragement and plan testing homework assignments for each other. Family members often need to be involved, especially if they have become part of the means of enabling the person to avoid fearful situations.

NURSING THE ANXIOUS PERSON

This chapter has so far considered the physiological signs and symptoms of anxiety, the psychological effects of anxiety, and some of the conditions that lead people to seek treatment. The ways in which nurses can help people who are suffering from disabling amounts of fear or anxiety will now be explored. It is rare for people suffering from these conditions to need to be admitted to hospital. Most are able to be treated as outpatients, in clinics, in day hospitals, or in their own homes. However, anxiety can often be seen among patients with long-term major mental illness who are faced with changes in their routine and among those suffering from what is diagnosed as an 'agitated depression'. People undergoing withdrawal programmes from alcohol or drug dependency frequently experience great anxiety. All these groups of people may need to be cared for in hospital for a period. The techniques used by nurses are equally applicable in the care of anxious people whether they are being cared for in hospital or in the community.

Nurse behaviour therapists undergo a post-registration course in which they learn, and practise under supervision, the skills and techniques of what is now called cognitive behavioural therapy. They learn to apply the theory of both cognitive therapy and behaviour therapy. It is rare now in the field of psychiatry that pure, behaviour modification techniques are used alone. For a more detailed description of the techniques used in cognitive behavioural therapy see Chapter 13.

Barker (1982), in the preface to his book *Behaviour Therapy Nursing*, opens by stating 'Nurses help people.' He goes on to say that there are occasions when, 'it is more appropriate merely to alleviate distress, or to encourage the acceptance of handicaps, than to strive too resolutely for the elimination of such problems'. People come for treatment, or 'help', because they are faced with difficulties in coping with the problems of life. Nurses can help by taking these problems of life seriously, listening to what people say, making a careful assessment of each person's life circumstances, identifying with each person just what exactly the problems are, and together working out what each person can do to bring about the changes that they wish in order for life not to be so problematical.

Community psychiatric nurses have found that many people are referred to them suffering from anxiety states which may have been very disabling to the individual for many years. Although they may not necessarily be fully qualified nurse therapists they are able to use the techniques of cognitive behaviour therapy to enable their patients and clients to learn ways of overcoming their fear and anxiety and of learning to cope better with the problems faced every day. Much of the success of these techniques has come about through rigorous testing in research, using scientific measures to evaluate the outcomes of treatment methods.

Throughout treatment the client and the nurse are partners, collaborating in the treatment programme at all stages. Together they use a number of rating scales to assess the level of anxiety in particular situations. It is important to establish a baseline from which the client and the therapist can measure progress. Together they identify the problems and agree which ones are to be tackled in therapy and which the client can deal with in homework exercises. They have to agree and learn to trust one another. If either is only half-hearted then the chances of success are greatly reduced. The person has to be *motivated* to want to change those behaviours which are causing the problem. This may well involve challenging their thoughts and beliefs about the world around them that they may have held for very many years, beliefs that they learned when very young and now have to be unlearned. The role of the nurse as therapist in this situation is to teach and educate the client to new ways of thinking about and perceiving the world, of accepting his place in the world and of behaving and reacting to that world in ways that are acceptable both to the individual and to the society in which that individual lives.

Examples of questionnaires used in making an assessment of someone suffering from anxiety are:

- Fear Questionnaire
- Fear Survey Schedules
- Social Anxiety Scales
- General Health Questionnaire
- Beck Anxiety Inventory
- Beck Depression Inventory
- Fear of Negative Evaluation Scale
- Agoraphobic Cognitions Questionnaire
- Problem Profile

In all of these questionnaires clients are asked to rate themselves on a scale measuring from 0 to any number up to, say, 10 to indicate the amount of fear or anxiety felt. The scale may be used to measure feelings before treatment begins as part of the initial assessment, before and after a specific treatment session, or used over a period of time to measure overall progress. (See Appendix D for examples of rating scales.)

STAGES OF TREATMENT

As the nursing process is based on a *problem-solving* approach, likewise the stages of any treatment programme for people suffering from anxiety are based on the four stages of the nursing process:

- *Systematic assessment* of the problems
- *Detailed planning* of the action programme
- *Graded implementation* of the agreed treatment programme

- *Thorough evaluation* at each stage of the treatment programme

Assessment

The importance of making a full and relevant assessment has been stressed several times throughout this book. When working with someone who is anxious, the nurse needs to gather enough information from the client and any relatives who have close contact with the client to clarify the lifestyle and particular circumstances of that individual client. Having obtained a general picture, the nurse will then need to concentrate on helping the client to define exactly what the problem or problems are. The 'referred problem' may be one thing, but through the process of assessment it is often discovered that other problems are revealed.

Let us take Mary, for example. Her referred problem was that she had panic attacks whenever she had to stand in a queue, at a bus stop or in a supermarket checkout. This resulted in her no longer going out and becoming more isolated at home. On careful questioning it became clear that the panic attacks were secondary to her feelings about her ability to cope in social settings where strangers may be present. She had always felt shy and insecure among a crowd of people, but the feelings had become more acute following an occasion when she had dropped her purse as a bus approached. She felt that the other people in the queue were laughing at her and saying, 'What a clumsy, useless creature she is, holding up the bus!' Her anxiety and panic attacks had become generalized on her feelings of her own inadequacy in social settings.

Having identified the problems, the nurse and the

client then assess how much of a problem each one is and compile a hierarchy of problem areas; in other words they *prioritize* the problems.

It is during the stages of assessment that the nurse may wish to use one or more of the various assessment tools available, such as the questionnaire mentioned above, in order to establish the baseline of the degree of anxiety experienced by the client.

Once the nurse has gathered a full personal, family, and problem history, and has agreed exactly what the problem areas are that the client wishes to change, they can go on to the next stage of the process.

Planning

At this stage the nurse will have to decide whether treatment should proceed on an individual basis or whether the client may benefit more from joining a group of people with similar problems (see Chapter 13). In a group the members can work together and provide each other with support, encouragement and inspiration to keep trying and to experiment in ever bolder situations. It may also be very useful to engage members of the family in therapy, especially if it has been discovered that they have inadvertently been colluding with the client by helping him to avoid the very situations that must now be faced.

In Mary's case where it was found that the feared situation was not so much queuing as any social situation, it may be agreed that joining a group of six or seven other people with a similar fear of social settings would be more beneficial, where they would all be involved in social skills training. Mary would be given opportunities to challenge and be challenged on her beliefs about herself and her perception of herself in social settings. Her fellow group members will support and encourage her to think differently about herself so that gradually she will build up confidence in herself, learn to be more assertive, and no longer feel panicky in society.

The treatment programme may include the following measures.

- Keeping a daily diary of the times the client feels anxious, identifying the 'automatic self-defeating negative thoughts' that precede the feelings of anxiety, such as: 'I feel anxious', 'I can't cope', 'I shall make a fool of myself'.
- Learning relaxation techniques that will reduce the tension created by 'anticipatory anxiety', or help control the feeling of panic when in a situation, such as controlled breathing, muscle relaxation, 'cue cards' which consist of sentences that admit the difficulty *plus* the thought that it is possible to cope with the feelings.
- Tasks to perform by deliberately facing the situation that is feared, by exposing oneself to the situation. This may be by a process of gradual desensitization or by going straight into the most feared situation, remaining in the situation until the feelings of anxiety or panic subside, which they will sooner or later, and repeating this until the feelings of anxiety come down to a manageable level.
- The nurse will plan to go through each step carefully with the client, preparing the client for what he may experience, modelling or role-playing satisfactory ways of coping in each situation, encouraging the client to imagine being in the situation first, perhaps, before actually going out and facing it.

- It is usual to set homework between treatment sessions, and these will be carefully planned and explained both before treatment starts and at each session.
- The client will be asked to keep careful, accurate records of all tasks tackled and regularly to complete rating scales of how he feels at the beginning and end of each task, so that he can monitor his own progress and the nurse can assess at each stage whether an alternative strategy may be more helpful. The plan can be changed at any time if both nurse and client feel a different approach may be more productive.

It is essential that the client and nurse both understand very clearly what is expected from each other at every stage of therapy. Once they have agreed the treatment programme, when it is to start, where and who will be involved, how often they will meet, then the programme can begin.

Implementation

This is putting into practice the treatment plan agreed together. The nurse may take an active part in the programme by accompanying the client for the first few attempts at each new situation, but the aim is for the client to be able to face each difficulty on his own, recognizing his own ability to cope with and control his feelings. He now learns that although the situations may be difficult, and although he may never be entirely free of anxious feelings, nevertheless he no longer has to avoid the situations but can face them and survive. The nurse's role throughout the implementation process is to encourage, teach, model, using whatever skills and techniques are most appropriate and useful to each individual, and always to give praise for the successful completion of each step.

Evaluation

Evaluation goes on all the time and at each session. This is documented through the rating scales so that both the nurse and the client can monitor progress and discuss whether there needs to be a change in approach or in the programme itself. In order to assess the long-term success of a treatment programme, it is useful to include at the outset the opportunity for follow-up evaluation at regular intervals, such as at three months, six months, one year after treatment has ended.

Whether the nurse is involved in helping patients in hospital or in the community, the principles of the nursing process will assist the nurse to approach the care of the anxious or fearful person in an organized and systematic manner. Through the assessment process the history of the problems giving rise to the feelings of anxiety is established. Through planning, the specific goals of treatment are agreed and how they are to be achieved. Through implementation the agreed tasks are tackled and evaluated as each step is completed.

As anxiety is such a common feature in people who present with mental health problems, nurses often find themselves working with other colleagues such as psychologists or occupational therapists in running relaxation groups, anxiety management groups, social skills groups, activities of daily living groups as part of a general acute admission ward programme. These skills should be included in all general psychiatric training programmes and nurses should be given every opportunity to practise and develop these skills, with supervision from more practised and experienced members of their multidisciplinary teams. Nurses are with patients in hospital over the 24 hours, day and night, and have excellent opportunities to help them to learn new ways of facing difficult and fearful thoughts and situations. There are a number of techniques they can use, based on modelling and encouraging the questioning of distorted beliefs and perceptions about the world, that will enable patients to feel better about the way they face life and how they see themselves in society. The nurse can help patients and clients to find an acceptable level of anxiety that does not cripple or disable or interfere with living and the enjoyment of life.

SUMMARY

Anxiety is a natural feeling and at times is an aid to survival. It is only when feelings reach such a level as to interfere with the ability to lead a normal life that people tend to present for treatment. Anxiety can be free floating and occur out of the blue, at any time of day or night, and give rise to feelings of panic, with observable effects on the body such as a pounding heart, rapid pulse, rapid breathing, increased perspiration, feelings of nausea, faintness, dry mouth. These feelings may be a consequence of previous experiences with accompanying thoughts of a negative, self-defeating nature, which become generalized into other aspects of the person's life. These thoughts then have a direct influence on behaviour, and experience reinforces the faulty un-satisfactorily learned response to a situation.

The nurse's role is to work together with each

individual person to help to identify exactly what the problem areas are, to agree a treatment programme that will enable the person to learn new and better ways of managing in those difficult situations so that the person understands what is happening and retains control of his feelings. The nurse uses skills and techniques that are research-based and known to be effective, using the nursing process to organize care.

REFERENCES

Barker PJ (1982) *Behaviour Therapy Nursing*. London: Croom Helm.

Beck AT (1976) *Cognitive Therapy and the Emotional Disorders*. New York: International Universities Press.

Garland A & Atha C (1992) Generalised anxiety disorder—a cognitive perspective. *Community Psychiatric Nursing Journal* **12**(3): 12–18.

Hawton K, Salkovskis PM, Kirk J & Clark DM (1989) *Cognitive Behaviour Therapy for Psychiatric Problems—A Practical Guide*. Oxford: Oxford University Press.

Marks IM (1978) *Living with Fear—Understanding and Coping with Anxiety*. New York: McGraw-Hill.

Meichenbaum D (1974) *Cognitive Behaviour Modification*. University Programs Modular Studies. New York: Plenum Press.

Chapter 12
Caring for the Person who is Aggressive

INTRODUCTION

One of the principal aims of this chapter is to assist the inexperienced nurse in her understanding of some of the various factors which may trigger aggressive responses in certain people. Equipped with this knowledge she will be more able to prevent whenever feasible—or at least reduce—the incidence of aggressive behaviour. A later section of this chapter will examine the nursing skills required when aggression cannot be averted, as well as the principles of care should violence become inevitable despite strenuous efforts by the nursing team to prevent it.

CAUSES AND PREVENTION OF AGGRESSIVE BEHAVIOUR

The popular idea of psychiatric hospitals is that of places where there is a great deal of aggression. This thought is often expressed by nurses who have never worked in a psychiatric setting. They are surprised to learn that there may be much more aggressive behaviour to be seen in Accident and Emergency Units—particularly at weekends.

The experienced nurse knows that physical aggression

is not common but acknowledges that impulsive behaviour sometimes occurs, though there is little real danger of physical injury. She may have forgotten, however, that:

- competence,
- self-assurance,
- skilled observation,
- special knowledge of the individual patient,
- ability to anticipate his responses, and
- timely and tactful management of potentially difficult situations

are all important factors in preventing aggressive behaviour, and that this could occur more frequently if the nursing team were less competent or more tactless or insecure.

But the new nurse often experiences fear and misgivings and this insecurity can be communicated to the person who, in the presence of an inexperienced staff member, may also become frightened and insecure. This in turn may cause the person to become aggressive.

Another trigger of patients' aggression is an impoverished social environment which gives rise to boredom and frustration: if in addition there is little or no opportunity for open and frank discussion of grievances, resentment builds up and can be expressed in hostility towards staff.

A person's disturbed state of mind may also contribute to aggressive responses. For example, someone with paranoid delusions or auditory hallucinations may react aggressively to a situation that is perceived as dangerous.

Sometimes aggression can be traced to disturbances in the relationship between people. Aggression, like anger, is not an attribute of a person, but a learned response to a frustrating or frightening experience. It is a feeling most people experience at one time or another.

Process of Control of Aggression

Children often express their aggressive feelings quite openly. When they are very young they kick and scream or have temper tantrums. As they grow older they learn to express their aggression more in speech and less in action, and later still, they learn to control their aggression. There are times when they give no overt indication of it at all.

In our society considerable value is attached to this process of control. In order to succeed in controlling aggression it is necessary, in the course of growing up, to experience it openly and to practise various methods of dealing with it. Children who are made to feel guilty about their aggressive impulses may lack practice in the process of control. Eventually they may succeed in hiding their aggression from everyone, even from themselves. They may appear meek and mild, gentle and placid. Behind this appearance may lurk the fear that to feel aggressive is dangerous and that any show of aggression might get out of control. It is possible that unconscious fear of their own aggression is to be found in nurses too. Possibly the fear many nurses express of being attacked by a patient is caused by anxiety that their own aggression might be aroused by such a patient.

It is a necessary stage in the control of aggression that one should be consciously aware of its existence. Children who have never been allowed to say that they felt angry with their parents are much more likely to have difficulty with their repressed aggressive feelings than those who in an angry moment can safely say to their parents 'I don't love you any more'. Some patients with aggressive tendencies have problems in exercising control over their behaviour. In the relative safety of a psychiatric setting patients' control may give way.

NURSING INTERVENTIONS

Helping the Person Control Aggression Responses

The patient's primary nurse, the person with whom he is most likely to have a therapeutic relationship, can sometimes take steps to avert an aggressive incident by picking up cues of tension, such as restlessness, pacing and distractibility. An effective nursing intervention may be a verbal acknowledgement of the patient's state of mind and an invitation by the nurse to talk things over; encouragement is given to the patient to ventilate his feelings. The nurse will listen attentively to whatever he has to say, without interrupting him and throughout the time the patient is speaking will maintain appropriate eye contact. Being listened to attentively is in itself therapeutic for a potentially aggressive person, as it is for any distressed person. Gradually he may be able to control his feelings. Clarification may be sought at some point if the reason for the person's anger is not apparent to the nurse.

Specific nursing interventions in the care of the aggressive person focus on helping him to learn methods of anger control and to learn new patterns of behaviour. These include therapy sessions which afford the patient the opportunity to consider, and sometimes role play, strategies that produce satisfying outcomes in the hope that they will gradually replace his customary aggressive responses to situations he perceives as provocative.

Nurses' Personal Reactions to Aggressive Behaviour

Nurses sometimes believe that it is wrong for them to experience anger or aggressive feelings. If a nurse tries to hide feelings of this sort, some of it may nevertheless manifest itself in actions such as:

- breaking things 'accidentally';
- making unnecessary noise;
- forgetting some attention promised to a patient; or
- avoiding altogether speaking to certain patients.

It is as necessary for nurses as it is for patients to feel free to talk about their frustrations and anger. Open discussion among colleagues at regular staff meetings is necessary to make sure that the needs of patients with aggressive tendencies are met without nurses losing control over their feelings. Prejudices and expectations will require to be explored. It may be that the nurse's own difficulties are a factor in the escalation of a potentially volatile situation.

Displaced Anger

The anger of an individual patient may not be directed against nurses personally. It may be aimed at his partner or mother and may arise whenever anyone unconsciously reminded him of the disliked person. The nurse may represent a 'parent figure' to the patient whose hostile feelings are then vented on the nurse. It helps a great deal to remember that in these cases the nurse 'stands for' someone else. If nurses learn not to take the patient's aggression any more personally than his affection, they can usually deal with the situation effectively. Frequent multidisciplinary team meetings for all those dealing with the patient are necessary in order to understand his attitude and so to be able to modify it.

The Deluded Person

Some people are angry about delusional frustrations. If the person thinks he is being poisoned he very understandably wishes to protect himself. It may not always be possible to predict impulsive behaviour if it arises from a delusional system or if it occurs in response to the command of 'voices'. But though it may not always be possible to predict when a deluded person will become angry, if the nurse knows him well it may be evident that an impulsive outburst may occur. If the nurse does not contradict or argue but reacts with empathy—tries to understand how things must appear from the patient's point of view—the patient's behaviour assumes a meaning. When it is appreciated that he acts as if his delusions were true—and they are true to him—it is easier to help him.

THE VERBALLY AGGRESSIVE INCIDENT

In any facility in which potentially aggressive patients are cared for, the occasional aggressive outburst can escalate and a disruptive incident may occur. The better the organization of nursing care, the fewer these incidents. When they do occur they must be dealt with quickly and effectively.

An incident is more likely to happen when the staff are not in agreement about the best approach to the patient, when they do not work as a team. Such divisions between staff divert attention from the important task of preventing aggression and of creating a therapeutic environment for the patient. Furthermore a study by

James (1990) identifies a positive correlation between the level of temporary (agency) staff and the number of such incidents recorded. The prevention of physical aggression requires the nursing team to ensure that 'there is a detailed individual assessment of the patients, close cooperation between multidisciplinary team members, attention to the methods of communication by the patient and clearly defined systems for decision making which allow the patient a degree of control' (Ritter, 1989).

The person who is using offensive and threatening language may respond positively to someone who is able to refrain from reacting to this situation with any hint of hostility. It is also important to avoid patronizing terms such as 'calm down': rather, talking quietly to the patient and listening with close attention to any reply may help to de-escalate the situation. Preferably the nurse should use negotiation: 'shall we sit down over here?', if appropriate to do so, and when seated, appropriate body language—a non-threatening open posture and the use of eye contact without actually staring at the person—can reinforce an empathetic approach. Disclosure at this point may be effective. An honest admission by the nurse that he or she is afraid of the patient's threat of physical violence, while still communicating to him that the situation can be controlled if necessary, is more congruent with present day caring attitudes than with the confrontational ('macho-image') stance sometimes associated—though not always justifiably so—with the custodial care of former years. The nurse's confidence is maintained in the knowledge that verbal intervention is part of a planned strategy by the nursing team as a whole.

THE VIOLENT INCIDENT

Nevertheless, despite the foregoing preventative measures, unexpected violence may still occur, and in order to meet the patient's needs and to ensure her own safety, the nurse must not act alone but summon aid immediately.

Highly skilled teamwork is essential to ensure that neither the patient nor the nursing staff are injured and that the safety of the other patients is not endangered.

Physical restraint may be required should the team leader's use of de-escalation skills fail. In settings where people with a potential for violent behaviour are cared for, the nursing team will preferably take part in in-service educational training to acquire the skills of control, restraint and disengagement (Turnbull *et al.*, 1990), or will have ready access to advice from a control and restraint nurse specialist.

Following a violent incident, the nurse concentrates on the need to build up the patient's shattered self-esteem by offering him a listening ear and non-judgemental, accepting responses to his words. Further nursing interventions aimed at improving the person's self-esteem form an integral part of his plan of care.

Documentation

Violent incidents must be promptly and accurately documented in accordance with managerial policy and a detailed account is also written in nursing records. Wright (1989) comments on a reluctance on the part of some nurses to record such episodes lest it reflects adversely on their professional practice. There ought to be no need for this concern provided management and members of the clinical team are supportive and show understanding towards their nursing colleagues.

Good nursing records are of value not only for assessment purposes should the patient be readmitted at any time, but also for providing details of nursing practices, antecedents of the incidents and other useful information such as staffing levels, time of day when the incident occurred and the staff members who were involved.

It is often hospital policy for the patient who has been involved in a violent episode to be examined by the doctor on duty even though the nursing team is confident that no injury has been sustained. This practice is a safeguard against any future litigation.

Post-incident Follow-up

Frequently the team leader remains with the patient after an aggressive or violent incident to afford him the opportunity, if he so wishes, to talk over what has happened; possible triggers may be identified and alternative modes of response examined. Each team member should also be given a chance to take part in a follow-up discussion afterwards and to evaluate his or her role in the incident.

Recent work by Whittington and Wykes (1989) and Farrell (1989) highlights the need of witnesses or victims of an aggressive or violent outburst to talk about their feelings and to discuss the precise details of the event; the student nurses questioned wanted their reactions to the event acknowledged in an empathetic manner by their ward colleagues. Recognition of the need for support, regardless of the degree of aggression involved, has resulted in the establishment of an 'Assault Support Team' in a North American psychiatric hospital (Dawson *et al.*, 1988). Meanwhile other disciplines this side of the Atlantic, for example social workers, are considering similar schemes designed to support colleagues who have been victims of aggressive acts.

CARING FOR THE PERSON WHO IS AGGRESSIVE IN THE COMMUNITY

Though the above discussion has focused mainly on the care of the person in hospital, most of the principles are equally applicable to the person who shows aggression in a community setting. CPNs frequently visit people at home, and often carry out an initial assessment in the home in order to learn more about the social circumstances that may be contributing to the mental health problems. If there is any possibility of an aggressive response by the patient, or from relatives, there should be arrangements within the service for the CPN to visit with another member of staff. It may be advisable to invite the patient and his family to come to a health centre or clinic where there are likely to be more people about, rather than to visit someone in the comparative isolation of a home. Although it has already been said that violent and aggressive episodes directed at staff are rare in psychiatry, it is essential that staff are protected from taking unnecessary risks, that there are sensible guidelines known to all staff, and that there are opportunities for nurses working in the community to learn 'breakaway techniques' in case they find themselves in difficult circumstances. However, it cannot be emphasized enough that all nurses should be taught the psychological skills of 'talking down' and defusing potentially aggressive incidents, using all the methods discussed earlier in the chapter.

CPNs working in deprived, inner city areas, where there is a great deal of resentment, unemployment and frustration, leading to feelings of hopelessness and despair, find that they need to work in pairs. The type of precautionary measures that these services encourage include:

- informing the base of where they are going and the expected timescale of the visit;
- arranging to phone in to the base at a specified time to reassure the rest of the team of their safety;
- carrying personal alarms;
- carrying mobile phones in case the public phones are out of action and it is not always appropriate to use patients' phones.

These precautions apply as well to CPNs working in isolated, rural areas, where access to help is even more remote. As has been mentioned before, possession of firearms is much more common than it used to be, so that nurses, in whatever setting, need to be confident in knowing what to do and how to behave in threatening circumstances. It is up to service managers to ensure that guidelines and policies are in place and that nurses have opportunities to refresh themselves in practice through training and refresher courses so that they feel confident and competent in dealing with aggressive incidents, whether in hospital or in the community.

SUMMARY

Aggressive behaviour and outbreaks of violence, though by no means an everyday occurrence in hospital- or community-based psychiatric settings, do occasionally happen. A knowledge of some of the factors likely to trigger such reactions can be of considerable value in achieving the goal of preventing or reducing their incidence.

No less important in the care of the person with a tendency to react aggressively are the skills practised by the nursing team to abort outbursts of aggression or to cope competently should such measures fail.

The crucial need for adequate numbers of nursing personnel to have specialized training in the management of care of a violent person must be stressed if injury to the person in need or to those offering skilled interventions is to be avoided at all times.

REFERENCES

Dawson J, Johnson M, Kehiayan K *et al.* (1988) Response to patient assault: a peer support programme for nurses. *Psychosocial Nursing and Mental Health* **26**: 8–15.

Farrell GA (1989) Responding to aggression: the role of significant others for student psychiatric nurses. *Nurse Education Today* **9**: 335–339.

James D (1990) Increased violence in an acute psychiatric ward. *Nursing Times* **86**(40): 54.

Ritter S (1989) *Manual of Clinical Psychiatric Nursing: Principles and Procedures*. London: Harper and Row, p. 83.

Turnbull J, Aitken I, Black L *et al.* (1990) Turn it around: short term management of aggression and anger. *Journal of Psychosocial Nursing* **28**(6): 7–10.

Whittington R & Wykes T (1989) Invisible injury. *Nursing Times* **85**(42): 29–32.

Wright B (1989) Threatening behaviour. *Nursing Times* **85**(42): 26–29.

SECTION IV: SPECIFIC THERAPEUTIC INTERVENTIONS

Chapter 13
Psychological, Physical and Social Interventions

INTRODUCTION

Nurses take part in a whole number of therapeutic interventions, whether these be to assist with the activities of daily living, to build up trusting relationships so that patients feel able to speak of their fears and troubles, or to undertake a specific intervention. In this chapter, the three main themes that have been followed throughout the book of psychological, physical and social aspects of care are taken separately and some specific interventions are considered in more detail. Psychological interventions are taken first as this is a book for psychiatric nurses whose chief difference from general nurses is their concentration on the mental health of their patients, or, in many cases, the mental illness of their patients.

Frequently, the success of psychological interventions depends on the concurrent physical interventions such as drug therapy, and, in severe cases of depressive illness, on electroconvulsive therapy, to lift or control the extremes of depression, and occasionally elation or thought disorder.

One of the consequences of most types of mental illness

is a loss of confidence, especially in social settings. Many people describe an inability to relate to others. They are unable to make or sustain relationships, and they lack the social skills that enable them to feel accepted and wanted by other people.

Some therapeutic interventions that nurses use, whether they are caring for their patients in the community or in hospital, are now described.

PSYCHOLOGICAL INTERVENTIONS

Counselling

Psychiatric nurses cannot call themselves counsellors unless they have undergone additional training, which will include receiving counselling for themselves from a trained and experienced counsellor and accepting supervision for the work that they do, either on an individual basis or in groups. However, as seen in Chapter 6, the skills that nurses are called upon to use when communicating with patients and their relatives are those that counsellors use in the more formal setting usually associated with counselling. These are the skills of *listening* and *responding*.

Counselling as a term has come to be used in many contexts, both within and without the caring professions. There are so many schools of thought and approach, developed from different contrasting theories, that counselling is in danger of being considered the panacea for all things. The foundation of counselling is in the work of people such as Freud, Jung and Adler. Their theories form the tools of psychoanalytical and psychodynamic therapies. From these beginnings, other people who were interested in what makes people think and behave in the way they do have explored human development and behaviour from different aspects. They have developed their own theories and approaches which have been adapted into clinical practice, and which can be simplified into two main groupings, the *behavioural approach* and the *person-centred approach*. The list of theories is long, and includes names like Abraham Maslow, with his theory of a 'hierarchy of needs' (see p. 73), Eric Berne who developed the theory of transactional analysis, based on child, parent, adult states and how they influence behaviour, Fritz Perls, who introduced gestalt therapy, Gerard Egan and Carl Rogers whose approach centres on the therapeutic relationship that exists between the client and the therapist, to name but a few.

It is beyond the scope of this book to describe in detail any of what have come to be called the 'talking therapies'. However, as already seen, psychiatric nurses spend much of their time talking with patients and with the relatives of the people in their care. This section of the book attempts to give a brief introduction to some of the principles and techniques common to most approaches to counselling and which nurses caring for people with mental health and emotional problems could learn to use in whatever setting they find themselves. They are centred around the two main areas of communication: the need to *listen* and the need to *respond*.

Listening Skills

Active listening involves the following.

- Giving full attention to what is being said—not allowing oneself to be distracted.
- Concentrating on what is being said—not allowing

one's own thoughts and feelings to get in the way of hearing what is being said.

- Observing the non-verbal signs, e.g.:
  - posture (slumped, upright, tense);
  - eye contact (present, avoided, fleeting);
  - facial expression (sad, angry, anxious);
  - action of hands (fidgeting, wringing);
  - position (close or distant);
  - breathing rate (rapid or relaxed).
- Clarifying what is being said by using a number of techniques.
  - Paraphrasing—restating what the client has said, either using the same words or using other words to express the client's thoughts and feelings, to check out that what the client said has been understood. It may often serve to summarize or express in a more concise and specific way.
  - Reflecting—repeating what the client has said, to check that it has been received and understood correctly.
  - Summarizing—restating and checking out the different issues, thoughts and feelings that have been expressed into a concise and specific framework. It can be done several times in a session and can be very useful when material brought up by the client is complex and difficult.
  - Questioning—'Open questions' are those that enable clients to expand and explore further the thoughts and feelings which have been touched on and often lead to clients making connections for themselves. 'Closed questions' are those that elicit a 'Yes/No' answer. They are only useful when seeking clarification of a specific point.
  - Challenging/confronting—drawing attention to inconsistencies, contradictions, avoidance or reluc-

tance in facing or admitting to the difficult parts of oneself and one's behaviour, or in experiencing the feelings that arise in the counselling process.

Responding Skills

- Warmth—the ability to show and feel acceptance and pleasure in the person's company, as being someone of worth and value and dignity.
- Genuineness—the ability to feel real and sincere interest in each person.
- Empathy—the ability to enter into the feelings of the other person, to acknowledge the reality of their feelings, to put oneself into the position of the other person and imagine how he or she must feel.
- Respect—to show that the counsellor truly respects the client as a distinct and whole individual.
- Non-judgemental attitude.

In addition the counsellor should develop the following qualities.

- The ability to allow individuals to identify and clarify their own thoughts and feelings, to become more self-aware and to develop the confidence to make their own decisions and become responsible for their own lives.
- The knowledge and ability to keep quiet or respond appropriately.
- An awareness and knowledge of how to handle transference and counter-transference in the counselling relationship with sensitivity and honesty.
- The ability to show tolerance and patience.
- The ability to recognize the limitations in what to expect, both from oneself and from the client.

- A sense of humour and to know when to use it.

Nurses may find themselves using these techniques in a variety of situations. These may include the formal situation when, as the primary nurse, a specific time has been set aside on a regular basis to explore together whatever issues have been identified as problem areas. There may be the more informal times when someone comes up to a nurse and says, 'Please may I talk with you', or 'I need to speak with someone now'.

As knowledge and skills have developed and evolved through practice and research, so it has become possible to predict which approach may be more likely to be successful with different groups of people presenting with certain problems. Each approach is focused in a different way.

- The psychoanalytic approach concentrates on the power of unconscious feelings and thoughts which can be accessed through 'free association', and on how early experiences which have been repressed can influence behaviour.
- The cognitive behavioural approach encourages the correction of faulty beliefs which have influenced the development of unsatisfactory ways of coping with life. The client is helped to identify and challenge negative automatic thoughts and assumptions and to replace them with positive statements that enable them to alter their perception of themselves and their environment. It is very clearly problem-oriented.
- The person-centred approach allows the client to express and explore feelings in such a way as to enable him to take full responsibility for himself and for the decisions that he makes, so that he achieves greater self-awareness, self-dependence and confidence.

Whatever the approach adopted there are several characteristics that are common to most of them which will now be considered.

People will usually seek help only when they become aware that something is not satisfactory with their lives. They may have a good idea of what that is, as in the case of a relationship that is breaking down, or they may only be aware that they seem unable to make a lasting, loving relationship at all. They may come to a counsellor hoping that the counsellor will solve the problem and make things better for them. Therefore, one of the first things to establish at the start of any counselling relationship is an understanding of the expectations of both the counsellor and the person seeking help.

The Counselling Process

Someone who is troubled in mind seeks help. This presupposes that the person seeking help has recognized that something is wrong, that they wish to find out what it is and do something about it. There needs to be a willingness to explore and change and grow, to take responsibility for one's decisions and actions, to become more self-aware, more self-accepting, more self-dependent and more confident.

The degree to which a person can achieve change and growth depends to a large extent on the therapeutic relationship that develops between the individual and the counsellor, and this will depend greatly on the initial impression created at the first contact and the transference (see below) that occurs between the individual and the counsellor. How the counsellor is able to use that transference to enable the individual to understand the relationships in his own life will influence the extent to which that person is able to change and develop more satisfactory ways of coping with life.

Transference is described as the process by which an individual perceives qualities and attitudes that belong to someone, usually a person from earlier experience, and attributes them to the counsellor or therapist or nurse. By being aware of this process the counsellor is able to assist the person to make the connections between past experience and feelings and present misperceptions and reactions which may result in continued unsatisfactory behaviour and responses. It is always an unconscious process, but by helping individuals to become aware of this process they are better able to understand their behaviour and change the way in which they interact with people.

In the same way the counsellor is made aware of the feelings and reactions aroused in him/herself by the individual. This is known as the *countertransference*. The counsellor helps the client to express in words and find meaning for the thoughts and feelings that have not been understood before; the client is able to make connections between thoughts, feelings and actions which have seemed inexplicable before, but, throughout the counselling process, gradually begin to make sense, leading to the client having the choice to take greater responsibility for his or her own life.

To summarize. The counselling process is that by which one person seeks out another in order to explore the inner world which governs thoughts, feelings and behaviour, usually with the aim of understanding and changing unsatisfactory aspects of that behaviour so that one is better able to cope with the difficulties that arise in life, one is able to make more satisfactory relationships and be responsible for one's decisions, by becoming more self-aware, self-confident and self-dependent. This may be achieved by the counsellor using the skills of listening and responding as the client explores that inner world.

Relaxation

Relaxation techniques have been recognized as a useful tool by behaviour therapists for many years. The ability to recognize tension and stress in oneself, coupled with the knowledge of how to lessen that tension gives back to people the sense of control that is frequently lost or feared by people who present with anxiety in any form. Teaching relaxation in isolation from specific applications can be of limited value, but by enabling people to recognize the triggers that cause tension and anxiety, and by equipping them with the means of reducing and controlling the degree of anxiety experienced, relaxation techniques have a useful place (see Chapter 11). The most commonly used technique is that of inducing muscle tension and relaxation as described by Jacobsen in the 1930s, by which the person is encouraged to examine the difference between a state of tension and a state of relaxation in the individual muscle groups of the body, and at the same time is taught to control the breathing.

Essential Components to Teaching Relaxation

- A quiet room.
- Space to lie on the floor on a comfortable rug or mattress with a pillow under the head, or a comfortable armchair that provides support to the head and arms.
- A warm, comfortable temperature.

- An allotted span of time that will be free of interruptions.
- Loose, comfortable clothing.
- An empty bladder.

Processes of Teaching Relaxation

- Work through each stage of the exercises with the person at the first session, demonstrating the areas with which the person has difficulty, before giving them an audiotape to play at home.
- Describe the exercises in detail and explain that it may take some practice before the benefits of the exercises are felt.
- Emphasize that regular practice at home is essential for any lasting benefit to be gained.
- Explain that although the initial learning of the techniques and the achievement of a state of relaxation may take 20–30 minutes, as practice progresses so the ability to reach a relaxed state and prevent tension and anxiety developing will become much quicker and easier.

Progressive Muscle Relaxation

Having set the scene and explained what is required of the patient and what the patient should expect the therapist talks the patients through the exercise:

Breathe normally through your nose at a slow, even pace. Now take a deep breath and hold it . . . now let it out slowly and study how your body becomes more relaxed.

We will now concentrate on the muscles of your hands and arms. First clench your right hand into a tight fist . . . study the tension in your right hand, study how it feels as the tension progresses up your right forearm . . . now let go and feel the difference as your right hand becomes relaxed. Now clench your left hand into a tight fist . . . study the tension as it progresses up your left forearm . . . now let go and feel the difference as your left hand becomes relaxed. Now hold your arms out in front of you and clench both your hands into tight fists . . . Feel the tension up both your forearms . . . Now let go and notice the difference as both your hands become relaxed. Shake your hands and let your fingers go limp.

Bend your elbows and tighten your biceps . . . Study the tension in your upper arms . . . now let go and feel the difference as your arms relax.

Hunch your shoulders up to your ears . . . Notice where you feel the tension . . . Study the tension . . . Now relax your shoulders and feel the difference as your shoulders become relaxed. Now hunch your shoulders towards your ears and circulate your shoulders, studying where you feel the tension . . . Now relax your shoulders. Let your head fall to the right . . . study the tension you feel in the left side of your neck . . . now let your head return to its normal position. Now let your head fall to the left and study the tension you feel along the right side of your neck. Let your head return to its normal position. Push your head hard into the back of the pillow (or back of the chair) . . . feel the tension in your throat and neck muscles . . . Return your head to its normal position. Drop your head forward onto your chest . . . Feel the tension in the muscles at the back of your neck . . . Relax your head to its normal position. Wrinkle your forehead and raise your eyebrows . . . Feel the tension in your face . . . Now relax your forehead. Open your eyes wide . . . relax . . . Shut your eyes, screw them tight, feel the tension around your eyes . . . Relax your eye muscles . . . Feel the difference as the muscles of your face relax. Clench your teeth . . . Study the tension in your jaw . . . relax. Push your tongue hard against the roof of your mouth . . . Notice the tension in your throat and tongue . . . Now relax. Take a deep breath . . . fill your lungs . . . hold it . . . now let your breath out slowly and as you breathe out feel how relaxed your body is becoming . . . Now breathe normally and slowly and comfortably.

We will now concentrate on the muscles of the rest of

your body. Take a deep breath and study the tension you feel in your chest . . . let your breath out and feel the difference. Pull in the muscles of your stomach tight . . . feel the tension in your stomach . . . study it . . . Now let go and feel the difference as your stomach becomes relaxed. Tighten the muscles of your pelvis and buttocks . . . study the tension . . . now let go and feel the difference as your pelvis and buttocks become relaxed. Stretch your toes up towards your knees and feel the tension in your calves . . . hold it . . . now let go and feel the relief as your legs relax. Stretch your toes towards the floor and feel the tension in your shins . . . Relax your toes.

We have worked through all the main muscle groups of your body. Lie back now (sit back) and breathe normally and naturally, allowing yourself to feel relaxed throughout the whole of your body. Remain there and enjoy the feeling of relaxation for two minutes . . . When I count up to three, open your eyes, have a good stretch and then sit up slowly. One-two-three . . .

Nurses and therapists adopt their own use of words and phrases. The above is an example of the principles of teaching progressive relaxation to people. Further examples of applied relaxation can be found in Hawton *et al.* (1989, pp. 92–96).

Anxiety Management

Anxiety management can be carried out either on an individual basis or in a group where the participants can give each other encouragement and support, and can see how, by persevering with the programme, they too can learn to control the feelings of anxiety and panic and bring them to manageable proportions. The principles remain the same whether the therapist sees the person in individual sessions or in group sessions.

Stages of an Anxiety Management Programme

1   Make a thorough assessment of each person's history including their problem history.
2   Together, with each person, identify the problem areas and place them in a hierarchical order, using rating scales to establish the degree of anxiety aroused by each situation.
3   Explain to each person the purpose of treatment, what together you hope to achieve, within a specific timescale, and establish that each person wishes to continue to engage in treatment.
4   Explain the psychological, physiological, behavioural and cognitive aspects of anxiety and their resulting effect on each person's experience.
5   Introduce a number of coping strategies which may include: relaxation techniques, distraction techniques, 'cue cards'.
    If using cognitive behavioural techniques each person is taught to identify and challenge automatic negative thoughts (see below).
6   Familiarize each person with the use of rating scales, questionnaires, keeping a daily diary of events, feelings and progress.
7   Agree a programme of addressing each anxiety-arousing problem area and begin 'in vivo' treatment.
8   Set 'homework' for each person to tackle between each session. If possible, encourage the assistance of spouse or partner as co-therapist, to enable and support the completion of homework tasks.
9   At the start of each session, go through the homework tasks to acknowledge achievement and effort, to establish where difficulties are still being experienced, before going on to other problem areas.

10 Evaluate progress at each session.
11 At the end of the agreed timescale evaluate whether there is a need to continue treatment for a further period or whether to terminate the treatment programme.

The above can only serve as an example of the processes involved in anxiety management. Any reader wishing to explore in greater detail the practical application of an anxiety management programme should refer to the manuals indicated in the References and Further Reading.

Behavioural Therapy and Cognitive Behavioural Therapy

Nurses became involved in treating patients along behavioural lines in the 1960s. The terminology used has varied from 'behaviour modification', through 'behaviour therapy', 'behavioural psychotherapy' to 'cognitive behavioural therapy', all of which reflects the evolutionary development of this aspect of psychological intervention. As more and more research was carried out into the effectiveness of using techniques that changed the way a person behaved in given circumstances, and more became known of the importance of the interplay between the unconscious thoughts and feelings experienced in the past and repressed in the memory, so the art and science of treating along behavioural lines has changed to take into account new knowledge and research findings. There has been a closer acknowledgement of the similarities and links between the behavioural approach and the psychodynamic approach to treatment (Hawton *et al.*, 1989).

In the introduction to their book *Behavioural Psychotherapy—A Handbook for Nurses* (1990), Richards and McDonald acknowledge the development of behavioural approaches as being an integral part of a psychiatric nurse's intervention skills, particularly useful to community psychiatric nurses who find the short-term, time-limited, problem-specific approach applies well to some of the people referred to them. Both basic and post-basic training programmes contain an element of teaching behavioural techniques and a growing number of nurses are choosing to become expert clinical specialists in the field of behavioural psychotherapy.

This section on specific intervention is only intended to introduce readers to the principles underlying these approaches. More detailed and specific texts are listed in the References and Further Reading.

The Three Systems Approach

Behavioural psychotherapy, or cognitive behavioural psychotherapy, as practised by nurses, provides an excellent illustration of the practical use of the nursing process framework:

- A thorough two-part *assessment* is made by which the nurse collects the information from which problems are identified.
- A treatment programme is *planned* and negotiated as a collaborative partnership between individual and therapist.
- This treatment programme is then *implemented* over a specified and agreed time scale.
- Outcomes of the treatment programme are *evaluated* at each session using rating scales by which both the

individual and the therapist can measure success and achievement.

The two part assessment consists of:

1   a problem assessment;
2   a general assessment.

Underlying all the information, the nurse is seeking to assess the effect problems have on three levels.

- Physiological—the effects of the problem on the autonomic nervous system.
- Behavioural—the way the problems affect the behaviour of the person.
- Cognitive—the thoughts and feelings experienced by the person when faced with the problems.

The problem assessment aims to assist the person to focus very specifically on the details of the problems, the frequency and intensity of their occurrence, the effect they have on behaviour and the consequences of that behaviour.

The general assessment looks at such areas as:

- mental state which includes:
  - general appearance,
  - behaviour,
  - conversation,
  - mood,
  - abnormal experiences,
  - memory and concentration,
  - sleep pattern,
  - appetite;
- past psychiatric and medical history;
- current social conditions;
- family history;
- personal history.

It is only once this very thorough assessment has been made that together the person and the therapist can begin to work out what has been attempted in the past, why perhaps it has not been successful and just what the individual person wants out of therapy at this particular time.

Treatment is not confined to the actual sessions with the therapist. The overall aim is to enable all individuals to learn that they can take control over themselves, that their symptoms do not control them. Much of the work is done between sessions in the form of homework tasks set during the session. Wherever possible the spouses or partners are encouraged to be involved in the treatment programme.

A daily diary is kept recording each stage of progress and before any new work is undertaken an evaluation of the previous work is made.

Forms are filled in and graphs are made illustrating the course of the treatment so that progress can be clearly identified and verified.

Cognitive Behavioural Therapy

The particular contribution to the development of behavioural psychotherapy made by people like Aaron Beck was the conviction that much that governs the way people behave in given situations is a consequence of early experiences which have become distorted and generalized into daily living so that assumptions are made which lead to unsatisfactory emotional and behavioural responses in similar situations.

Beck (1976) developed a system by which people are actively taught and encouraged to identify what he calls *negative automatic thoughts* and then systematically to challenge them. His *negative cognitive triad* looks at three areas:

1   the self,
2   current experience,
3   the future,

and examines how people regard themselves in each area.

For example, a woman suffering from depression may say:

1   I'm useless.
2   Nothing I do ever turns out right.
3   I will never feel any better.

As treatment progresses she will be gently encouraged to challenge each of these statements through her own experience by looking at successful achievements and recognizing the feelings experienced when she accomplished something that did turn out right. This will then be brought into the present so that she can acknowledge that she has achieved something, is therefore not useless but is competent, and this looks good for the future, replacing her previous feelings of hopelessness and despair with hope and a sense of direction and purpose.

Once again, the main aim of using a cognitive approach to treatment is to enable people to regain control over their own lives, to help them to identify what has gone wrong, when and how they have developed unsatisfactory ways of reacting to life's events, and teaching them alternative strategies based on more accurate assumptions, tested out by their own experiences. It is an approach based on problem-solving, by which everything is made explicit. It is time-limited. The person and the therapist work collaboratively, planning strategies together to deal with clearly identified problems towards explicitly agreed goals (Hawton *et al.*, 1989).

The process is the same as for behavioural psychotherapy.

- A detailed assessment is made of current difficulties.
- Aims of treatment are identified and goals defined.
- The concept of a vicious circle of negative thoughts and their consequences is explained.
- Treatment programme is planned and homework agreed.
- At each session a review of the previous session and feedback on the events of the intervening period are evaluated before starting on any new work.

Much of the initial work will be learning to identify the *negative automatic thoughts* that pop into one's head without any effort and then to identify the response to those thoughts. Frequently it will be found that they have become distorted and do not fit the facts, but they have become involuntary and serve to keep reinforcing the unhelpful and demoralizing attitude to oneself.

The treatment will be in learning to challenge these thoughts and testing out the truth or falsehood of the assumptions held over the years. Again it is a part of treatment to keep an accurate record of progress by using either a daily diary or record sheet to keep account of each stage of treatment. The relationship between a thought, a task, the feelings associated with the thought and task, are all closely monitored and examined.

PHYSICAL THERAPY: ELECTROCONVULSIVE THERAPY (ECT)

Introduction

The therapeutic properties of electricity can be traced back to the writings of Hippocrates. It was not until 1938, however, that Ugo Cerletti, an Italian neuropathologist, first used it to treat mental disorders by passing an electrical current between electrodes on each side of the head to induce a generalized seizure. This procedure known as electroconvulsive therapy (ECT) may be described as a therapeutic dose of electricity applied to a person's head, resulting in a convulsion. Modern ECT machines minimize the amount of current applied by the use of brief pulses lasting 1–2 milliseconds. Despite psychiatrists having used this treatment regularly for over the past fifty years it remains controversial.

Among the main objections raised by those who are opposed to ECT are:

- its mode of action is uncertain;
- it has harmful effects on the recipient's brain cells;
- it is a barbaric method and its use is degrading for the patient.

Some nurses have also felt that as in the right of conscientious objection to abortion they should be allowed to 'opt-out' when a patient in their care was prescribed a course of ECT. The National Board for Nursing, Midwifery and Health for Scotland (NBS) issued a Guidance Paper in September 1985 in which they state that the comparison with abortion 'is not a valid one' (p. 1). The NBS also state that the criticism that the administration of ECT is 'crude, dangerous and degrading is an emotionally loaded objection. Any surgical intervention could be described in similar terms' (p. 2).

One of the most controversial issues related to ECT centres on the important question: do its beneficial effects outweigh its risks?

Writing half a century after ECT was first used, two psychopharmacologists help to provide an answer when they assert that 'ECT still remains the most effective form of antidepressant treatment for severe cases of depression' (Silverstone & Turner, 1988). Carefully controlled trials confirm that ECT effects a significant therapeutic response in severely depressed patients, particularly in those who are *deluded* (Johnstone *et al.*, 1980; Gregor *et al.*, 1985). Addressing the question of adverse effects of ECT, Rose (1988) states that 'there is no evidence from either clinical studies or relevant animal investigations that ECT causes structural brain damage or is associated with the development of spontaneous seizures. Equally in general ECT does not appear to cause memory difficulties after the end of treatment' (p. 184). Any major complications or deaths associated with ECT usually occur in those people whose severe cardiorespiratory disease is adversely affected by the general anaesthetic given prior to the application of the electrical stimulus. (A course of treatment comprises approximately 6–10 ECTs given twice-weekly; the total number depending on individual patient response). This part of the chapter will discuss: (1) the indications and contraindications; (2) the possible mode of action and (3) the nurse's role in relation to the administration of ECT.

Indications and Contraindications

In addition to severe psychotic depression already mentioned, ECT is of value if severe depression is not responding to antidepressant drugs and also in women who become seriously mentally disturbed after childbirth. Very occasionally ECT may be the only effective form of treatment for the overactive and elated person who is resistant or hypersensitive to drugs (Carr *et al.*, 1983).

Absolute contraindications are few and may require to

be set aside for the person who is likely to come to serious harm if, due to his severe depressive state, he is refusing all food and drink. A recent history of cerebrovascular accident or myocardial infarction is usually included in the contraindications to ECT. The rationale for such caution is associated with the transient physiological changes known to occur with the passage of the electrical current and include:

- a considerable, though brief, increase in cerebral blood flow, with a concomitant sharp increase in blood pressure (systolic); and
- an initial bradycardia followed immediately by a short-lived but sudden tachycardia.

Neither the patient with epilepsy nor someone with a cardiac pacemaker needs to be excluded from a course of ECT. Extreme old age is not a contraindication (see also below).

Mode of Action of ECT

The exact mode of action of this form of therapy is unknown and this is a criticism put forward by those who object to its use. The National Board for Scotland point out, however, that 'the criticism that nobody knows precisely how ECT works is invalid in so far as in all areas of medicine proven and effective treatments are used before their precise action is known' (NBS, 1985, p. 2).

Research has confirmed that the successful application of ECT depends on the induction of a generalized seizure while animal studies have demonstrated wide-ranging effects on the activity of various chemical neurotransmitters (e.g. serotonin) and the sensitivity of their receptors in the brain.

The Nurse's Role

The care of the person for whom ECT is prescribed (usually by a consultant psychiatrist) may be divided into four stages.

1 Preparation for ECT.
2 Immediate care on the day of treatment.
3 Care during the procedure.
4 Care after the procedure.

Physical Preparation and Consent to Treatment

A thorough physical examination is carried out by a doctor to make sure the person is physically fit for the series of general anaesthetics involved in a course of ECT and for the treatment itself. A chest X-ray and, if required, an electrocardiogram (ECG) may be ordered. The nurse will record the patient's vital signs the evening before and again on the morning of treatment.

A full and clear explanation of the nature of ECT is given by the psychiatrist. It is vital that the patient is able to understand what is involved in the procedure and is given the opportunity to ask questions. A written summary may supplement the verbal explanation. Only after this has been done is the patient asked to give his written consent (see Appendix B for the relevant legal requirements if the patient is unable to give informed consent). Should the patient choose to withdraw his consent later, a member of the medical staff is contacted and the treatment deferred in the meantime. Relatives may be initially apprehensive when told that the patient is to have this form of treatment. They too should be given an explanation of what is involved and the opportunity to ask questions.

Sometimes a person who is severely depressed may—because of poor concentration—retain little or nothing of the information the doctor has given him. It can be helpful if the nurse takes advantage—if applicable—of the patient's diurnal mood variation (worse in the morning, slightly better towards evening) to repeat the doctor's explanation.

Although there are variations in the details of the explanation given to the patient, with some points stressed more than others, general principles are similar. It can be reassuring for the patient to be told, for example, that a member of the nursing staff (preferably his primary nurse) will accompany him to the ECT suite/clinic and will remain with him till fully recovered. It is also explained that the procedure is painless; a light anaesthetic is given by injection before a small amount of electricity is passed between electrodes placed on the head.

The patient is told that he will probably feel rather lightheaded on wakening from the anaesthetic for a brief period and that any headache or memory difficulties will be equally transient. A person about to have ECT for the first time can often benefit from the special attention of his primary nurse on the evening before treatment. She will devote time to repeat if necessary exactly what is involved and allow ample time for questions. This may be an ideal opportunity to correct any misconceptions the patient may have from the often inaccurate and sensational media coverage given to this procedure in the past.

To ensure an objective account is given to the patient it is important that the nursing staff are fully conversant with the latest literature/research on this topic. If a nurse should feel unable to give objective and accurate information it is important that she delegates this to someone who can.

A fellow patient who has previously benefited from

this form of therapy may be available and willing to spend some time with the apprehensive 'first-time' patient: this unique reassurance is invaluable.

Immediate Care of the Patient before ECT

However carefully the patient is prepared psychologically beforehand, on the day of his *first* ECT some apprehension is not unusual. Subsequent treatments engender much less fear and may be 'even pleasant' for some people (Gray, 1983). Meanwhile the nurse must do all she can to alleviate the patient's anxiety and continue to offer support until the patient is under anaesthesia in the treatment room.

The anaesthetist will request that the patient has neither food nor drink for a specified period of time before treatment is due and as is the practice before any general anaesthetic is administered, these instructions must be strictly followed. If any patient inadvertently has anything by mouth this must be reported immediately and the anaesthetist's instructions followed.

Final preparations include an explanation to the patient of the reasons why loose clothing is required (might restrict breathing) and why make-up or nail varnish is not worn (ensures accurate post-treatment observations of patient's colour); metal objects such as earrings and hairclasps are not worn in case they deflect the current; wedding rings may occasionally have to be secured if the person has lost a great deal of weight due to severe depression. Any other jewellery should be kept in a safe place until after the person has fully recovered. An identity bracelet is usually worn.

Immediately before leaving the ward the patient is

asked to empty his bladder to prevent incontinence due to the muscle relaxant which follows the anaesthetic.

Relevant documents collected by the nurse accompanying the patient include:

- a note of the patient's vital signs and current medication;
- ECT/consent form(s);
- the patient's case notes with any X-rays and results of investigations.

Electroconvulsive therapy is usually carried out in a central treatment facility. The trained nurse in charge of the clinic ensures that all the essential equipment is available and in working order and is responsible for reordering of any drugs required by medical staff. The nurse plays an important part in liaising with the ward staff concerning the approximate times of the treatment sessions and of any untoward delays which may occur.

Care of the Patient during Treatment

While in the waiting area, the nurse remains with the patient, guiding conversation and if appropriate providing distraction from the topic of ECT. In the treatment room, after introductions, the patient is asked to remove his footwear and to loosen any tight clothing before lying down comfortably on the trolley. Dentures (also any prostheses), if worn, are placed in a labelled container. The anaesthetist enquires about loose teeth and crowns; dislodged teeth may be inhaled during treatment. The blanket used to cover the patient should not extend over his feet so that any twitching of the toes may be clearly observed—this is sometimes the only sign that a convulsion has taken place.

The nurse continues to give the patient support until the anaesthetic has taken effect. After the anaesthetic and muscle relaxant are given (the muscle relaxant modifies the convulsion but must be given after the anaesthetic to prevent the patient being frightened by the distressing experience of being unable to breathe) oxygen is delivered by mask to inflate the temporarily paralysed lungs.

The nurse may be asked to gently immobilize the patient's limbs before the psychiatrist administers the current—each individual responds differently to the drugs and the electrical stimulus.

After the immediate effects of the passage of the electricity have ceased, the patient's lungs are again oxygenated until spontaneous breathing returns. As soon as the anaesthetist is fully satisfied that the patient is breathing independently an oropharyngeal airway may be inserted, the patient is carefully turned on his side in the recovery position, then taken to the recovery room—within earshot of the anaesthetist—to regain consciousness.

Care of the Patient after Treatment

The immediate aftercare of the patient follows the same principles as for anyone recovering from a general anaesthetic. The nurse in charge of the recovery room ensures beforehand that all resuscitation and suction equipment is in full working order. Until the patient is fully awake he is carefully observed and his vital signs are taken as instructed.

On recovery the patient will be confused, not knowing where he is or aware that he has had his treatment. His orientation will include the nurse talking clearly and slowly, calling him by name and reintroducing herself and anyone else present. After about 15 minutes or so the patient is helped to get up, tidy his hair and clothing, replace dentures etc., and assisted to the post-recovery area. Tea or coffee is offered and a light snack may be given now if the patient wishes or on return to the ward area. Information is again repeated as often as is necessary until the transient confusion clears; this may take slightly longer if the person is elderly. He will need to be reassured that this is only a temporary side-effect of the treatment. On return to the ward the patient may wish to lie down for a short period and a mild analgesic is offered if a headache is present.

The patient's mood and behaviour undergo considerable change during a course of treatment and these should be carefully observed and reported. One example, mentioned earlier (see p. 134) concerns the improvement in motor retardation which precedes any elevation of the patient's depressed mood and often occurs after the first few ECTs. The patient is now more active and able to carry out any suicidal plan he may have worked out during the apathetic and lethargic phase of his illness. Vigilance is not relaxed until the patient's mood also begins to show substantive signs of improvement.

A few patients may show an upward mood swing towards an abnormally elated state after several ECTs. After psychiatric assessment of the patient's mood further treatment may be postponed for the time being.

Outpatient ECT

Electroconvulsive therapy may occasionally be given to a person living at home and attending as an outpatient. An example may be someone who is unwilling to remain in hospital though his course of ECT and recovery is as yet incomplete.

Information is given to the patient and his relatives concerning the need to fast on the day of ECT, and also the date and time to attend the clinic. Other details include the necessity for the patient to be accompanied home after treatment—he must not drive—and to report any untoward side-effects to his GP or to the hospital. Alcohol should not be taken for the rest of the day to avoid any drug interactions; neither should the patient climb ladders nor use any power tools.

Before leaving for home the nurse in charge will ensure that the patient is fully recovered and has taken a light snack.

ECT and the Elderly Person

People with severe depression in later life have for some-time been regarded as good candidates for ECT and may respond better than those in younger age groups. Benbow (1989) and Murphy (1989) have found, however, that the elderly person may require a longer course before therapeutic effects are apparent. Brandon (1986) asserts that ECT is safer than most antidepressant drugs for the elderly person who has coronary heart disease; he also found that its therapeutic effects were more rapid than drugs—an advantage in all age groups.

SOCIAL SKILLS THERAPY

This section looks at some of the situations and problems that people frequently present with that prevent or interfere with normal social intercourse. Many of the techniques used by therapists are based on those already discussed—problem solving, systematic desensitization, anxiety management, relaxation, challenging self-defeating thoughts. Patients and clients are asked to identify the areas of social deficit, or in the case of people with long-term, institutionalized behaviour patterns, areas that are identified by staff after discussion with the patients, and treatment programmes are designed specifically to address those areas of behaviour that are unacceptable to the person, the family or society. Detailed descriptions of social skills treatment programmes can be found in many of the texts that deal with behaviour therapy.

The types of behaviour that are most frequently named include:

- lack of assertion—whether at home with family members, at work with colleagues or superiors, in social situations such as parties, in the pub, in shops, in groups where people are having discussions or informal conversations, with any interpersonal relationship;
- inability to control outbursts of anger or irritation;
- antisocial behaviour such as interrupting other people's conversation, failure to recognize when it is inappropriate to invade individual personal space, asking for money, cigarettes, etc., passivity;
- neglecting one's self-care, hygiene, appearance;
- fear of eating and drinking in public places.

Nurses and therapists used to run groups under the broad heading 'Social Skills Training Groups', in which they attempted to draw together small groups of people who described or exhibited behaviour considered to be socially undesirable. It is more the custom nowadays to give the groups specific titles which more nearly describe the skill that is being addressed, e.g.:

- assertiveness training;
- anger management;
- daily living skills training.

It has usually been found that most people benefit from treatment, training, education, whichever emphasis is most acceptable, in a group setting, although some people find this too threatening at first. With those people it may be more useful to start with a few individual sessions before introducing them to a group or building a group around them. The benefits of group settings for social skills therapy are that the group members are able to support and encourage each other, share ideas and experiences, measure their own progress and development against each other, have more people on which to model their own behaviour and learn what is socially appropriate behaviour in a variety of situations.

Whatever the diagnosis of the condition, many people suffer an accompanying degree of anxiety. This is often overlooked in the case of people with psychotic illnesses whose delusions and hallucinations may add to their lack of confidence. The feelings of anxiety can lead to social withdrawal and a subsequent poor quality of life which may affect not only the individual patient or client, but other members of the family as well. This anxiety may be due to an inability to assert oneself in an effective way.

Assertiveness must not be confused with aggressiveness. One is the ability to relate to other people in an appropriate manner that is acceptable to all parties concerned; the other is to express feelings in an inappropriate manner that is not socially acceptable. To be assertive takes into account the feelings of other people; to be aggressive does not. Most of us find it difficult to say no to people on some occasions and feel annoyed with ourselves when we feel we have been weak or allowed ourselves to be manipulated, or have agreed to something we knew we would be unable to honour. Instead of saying, 'I am very sorry but I am unable to do that for you', or 'I am sorry but I disagree with you about that', we find ourselves agreeing, either because we cannot face a disagreement or argument or because we do not want to disappoint the other person.

Shyness is more often than not due to anxiety that arises from a lack of confidence in social situations. People feel uncomfortable when they have to speak to others. They cannot think what to say or how to behave. This may be due to an unrealistic desire always to appear clever, witty, outgoing, friendly and to be liked by everyone all of the time. Any lack of the wished-for response can be interpreted as failure and give rise to increasing levels of debilitating anxiety to such an extent that the person withdraws from any social situation and so tries to avoid feeling the anxiety.

In all treatment programmes in which the patient and therapist seek to change or modify unsatisfactory behaviours the same principles apply.

1   Identify the behaviours that are unsatisfactory.
2   Agree the desirable goals to be achieved.
3   Explain the processes by which they will be achieved.
4   Set small steps that are easily achieved first.
5   Agree a system of review and evaluation.

The stages that constitute assertiveness training

- Understanding the different elements of communication.
- Introducing oneself.
- The use of 'small talk' in developing a conversation.

- Knowing why you wish to speak to someone, what you wish to say.
- Conveying meaning through the way one speaks:
  - tone of voice;
  - speed of speech;
  - length of speech.
- The significance of non-verbal behaviour:
  - eye contact;
  - body language—posture;
  - facial expression;
  - position;
  - gesture.

The emphasis in assertiveness training is on building up confidence and self-assurance through positive feedback at every stage, acknowledging effort and progress so that people are able to think well of themselves and their abilities. In a group setting it is best to have two therapists who use themselves to model different behaviour strategies initially. Much of the subsequent work will be based on roleplay, with the members of the group practising how to deal with different situations and with different people, e.g.:

- young man introducing himself to a girl at a party, in the pub, at work and so on;
- girl saying 'no' to unlooked-for approaches from member of opposite sex;
- daughter exerting her own wishes over a domineering mother;
- employee seeking a rise in salary at work;
- taking a damaged article back to a shop;
- negotiating a loan from bank manager;
- telling one's spouse one no longer wishes to spend every Sunday with the in-laws.

At each session homework exercises and targets are set for the members of the group to practise their new skills and gain confidence. These are reported back to the group at the start of each session and positive feedback given for effort and achievement. New skills are practised at each session and new exercises given of increasingly challenging situations until either the agreed number of group sessions is reached or the individual has achieved the original goals set.

SUMMARY

This chapter has illustrated a few of the specific therapeutic interventions that nurses working in the mental health field will be using, whether the focus of their work is in a hospital setting, an outpatient clinic, a day centre or in the patient's own home. It is not an exhaustive list, nor has it attempted to apply the interventions on every appropriate occasion. Frequently all three levels of intervention may well be necessary, psychological, physical and social, in order to treat a person's illness, assist in changing unsatisfactory behaviours and enable that person to live a more meaningful life or raise the quality of life.

Relationships and relating to other people are central to our existence as human, thinking, feeling beings. How we talk to each other, how we behave towards each other, how we express what we feel for each other, all influence how successfully we are able to function in society. People become mentally ill when these processes no longer work for them. Nurses play an important part, along with their colleagues from other professional backgrounds and, in particular, by acknowledging the role of family and relatives, in helping these people to regain their peace of mind or learn new ways of living more fulfilling lives.

All the interventions described have both a 'talking' element and a practical element. All require to be explained fully to the patient to gain cooperation and to identify what exactly it is that the patient wishes to achieve. Often the patient expresses this by saying 'I only wish to feel better'. By using a combination of physical treatments to combat the extremes of emotion experienced by people, plus psychological treatments to assist in understanding why feelings arise and social skills training to modify behaviour that is generally unacceptable to society, this can be achieved.

FURTHER READING

Brooking J, Ritter S & Thomas B (eds) (1992) *A Textbook of Psychiatric and Mental Health Nursing*. Edinburgh: Churchill Livingstone.

Egan G (1993) *The Skilled Helper*. Belmont: Brooks-Cole.

Fraser M (1982) *ECT: A Clinical Guide*. Chichester: Wiley.

Nelson-Jones (1988) *The Theory and Practice of Counselling Psychology*. London: Cassell.

Noonan E & Spurling L (1992) *The Making of a Counsellor*. London: Tavistock/Routledge.

Rogers C (1961) *On Becoming a Person*. London: Constable.

Simpson K & Oswald A (1994) Anaesthesia for ECT. In: Gibson H (ed.) *Psychology, Pain and Anaesthesia*. London: Chapman & Hall.

Williams M (1992) *The Psychological Treatment of Depression. A Guide to the Theory and Practice of Cognitive Behaviour Therapy*. London: Routledge.

REFERENCES

Beck A (1976) *Cognitive Therapy and the Emotional Disorders*. New York: Penguin.

Benbow S (1989) The role of ECT in the treatment of depressive illness in old age. *British Journal of Psychiatry* **155**: 147–152.

Brandon S (1986) The treatment of depression. *British Medical Journal* **292**: 288.

Carr V, Dorrington C, Schrader G & Wale J (1983) Use of ECT for mania in childhood bipolar disorder. *British Journal of Psychiatry* **143**: 411–415.

Gray E (1983) Severe depression: a patient's thoughts. *British Journal of Psychiatry* **143**: 319–322.

Gregor S, Shawcross C & Gill D (1985) The Nottingham ECT study. *British Journal of Psychiatry* **146**: 520–524.

Hawton K, Salkovskis P, Kirk J & Clark D (1989) *Cognitive Behaviour Therapy for Psychiatric Problems—A Practical Guide.* Oxford Medical Publications.

Jacobs M (1982) *Still Small Voice—An Introduction to Pastoral Counselling.* London: SPCK.

Jacobs M (1985) *Swift to Hear—Facilitating Skills in Listening and Responding.* London: SPCK.

Johnstone E, Lawler P, Stevens S, Deakin J, Frith C, McPherson K & Crow T (1980) The Northwick Park ECT Trial. *Lancet* **ii**: 1317–1320.

Murphy E (1989) Depression in the elderly. In Herbst K & Paykel E (eds) *Depression: An Integrated Approach.* Oxford: Heinemann Medical Books.

National Board for Nursing, Midwifery and Health Visiting (1985) Guidance Paper. National Board Scotland.

Nurse G (1980) *Counselling and the Nurse.* Aylesbury: HM+M Publishers.

Richards D & McDonald R (1990) *Behavioural Psychotherapy—A Handbook for Nurses.* Oxford: Heinemann Nursing.

Rogers C (1978) *Carl Rogers on Personal Power.* London: Constable.

Rose N (1988) *Essential Psychiatry.* Oxford: Blackwell Scientific Publications.

Silverstone T & Turner P (1988) *Drug Treatment in Psychiatry.* London: Routledge and Kegan Paul.

SECTION V: LOOKING AHEAD

Chapter 14
Challenges for the Future

INTRODUCTION

This book has attempted to describe mental health nursing both in its historical context and where it is at present, and has given examples of the kind of situation and practice that students new to mental health care may find themselves in when they begin their experience, either in a hospital setting or in the community.

This final chapter introduces some of the issues facing mental health nurses in the 1990s, issues which must influence the way in which care is delivered to people with mental health problems. In their turn these will influence the type of training and preparation to care which responds to the needs of people with mental health problems and of families and other carers who carry the main burden of care outside hospitals.

THE POLICY CONTEXT

Mental health nursing is faced with responding to policy decisions that have huge implications, not only in the field of nursing practice, but clearly in the realms of pre- and post-registration training, education and research.

These policy decisions include directives coming from the wider European Union context as well as those from within the British Government and nursing itself. The Department of Health (1992) announced its health strategy for England in *The Health of the Nation* document, in which one of its five priority areas is mental health, which includes reduction in the number of suicides by the year 2000. It has set up a Mental Health Task Force to facilitate initiatives to improve the care of people with mental health problems. Alongside all the Government initiatives that have been announced in recent years is the Department of Health's strategy for nursing *A Vision for the Future*, launched in April 1993.

The Patient's Charter (Department of Health, 1991) encourages the empowerment of patients with their right to information and has set national standards with the intention that all services expand these by developing their own local Charters.

The NHS and Community Care Act 1990 set guidelines for the provision of care and demanded evidence that the needs of people with severe mental disorder are being adequately considered and met. Arising from the deep concern expressed by carers and from recent incidents which highlight the gaps in the provision of care in the community for people with severe mental illness, the Government is again considering whether to introduce new legislation in the form of Community Supervision Orders.

Specific areas of concern have been highlighted such as the plight of the homeless, so many of whom have mental health problems, the needs of people from ethnic communities which are not being met, the proper provision for people with mental health problems who find themselves in prison instead of receiving treatment and care for their mental disorder.

All services need to pay considerable attention to examining how well they are responding to need in their areas. They should be setting standards of care and measuring their outcomes through regular audit, on a multi-disciplinary basis as well as on a single professional basis.

All these issues and developments will have been considered by the Mental Health Nursing Review set up by the Department of Health, under the chairmanship of Professor Tony Butterworth in 1992. The report on its findings will be of crucial significance to the future of mental health nursing in Britain.

HEALTH OF THE NATION

In its White Paper *The Health of the Nation* (Department of Health, 1992) mental health is one of the five priority areas identified by the Government. The targets are:

- to improve significantly the health and social functioning of mentally ill people;
- to reduce the overall suicide rate by at least 15% by the year 2000 (from 11.1 per 100 000 population in 1990 to no more than 9.4);
- to reduce the suicide rate of severely mentally ill people by at least 33% by the year 2000 (from the estimate of 15% in 1990 to no more than 10%).

To achieve these targets mental health nurses along with their colleagues in the community nursing services will need to pay attention to the significance of poor housing options for people, employment opportunities with the stress that accompanies redundancy, the difficulties of returning to work after a period of absence particularly following mental breakdown, and the problems facing people with continuing mental illness in being accepted by the community. Factors which are known to contribute to an increase in mental health morbidity such as unemployment and poverty play an even more significant part in exacerbating the difficulties of people with severe mental health problems. How will psychiatric nurses meet the apparent contradiction posed by the squeeze on public spending and achieving the targets set above?

Nurses will need to develop their skills in assessing suicidal risk and in recognizing the signs that may lead to suicide attempts, particularly among the more vulnerable groups that have been identified, such as young men, and in particular, suicide among the elderly and those who have severe mental illness. The challenge for mental health nurses will be in working within multidisciplinary teams to respond to the needs of the most vulnerable and disabled members of the communities they serve in such a way as to achieve the Department of Health's objective 'To reduce ill-health and death caused by mental illness' (Department of Health, 1992).

THE PATIENT'S CHARTER

The Patient's Charter has made explicit many of the rights that already existed, such as number 5: 'To be given a clear explanation of any treatment proposed, including any risks and any alternatives, before you decide whether you will agree to the treatment'. Nurses have frequently felt constrained as to their freedom to explain reasons for treatment to patients, having been told emphatically that that is the role of their medical colleagues. They now have an equal role in ensuring that patients and their carers are given as much information as they wish and require.

The other main contribution of the Patient's Charter is to introduce the notion of National Standards which must be measured and reported on regularly. Such standards as number 1, 'Respect for privacy, dignity and religious and cultural beliefs' have implications for the treatment of people from ethnic minorities and calls into question many common practices which nurses will need to reconsider. How often do nurses actually check out how each person wishes to be addressed? How familiar are all nurses with the cultures of all the people that they visit in the community or who come into hospital? Do all nurses know where to contact the religious leaders of each group within their communities?

Discharge Planning

Number 9: 'Discharge of patients from hospital' raises issues that patients, and especially their carers, have been concerned about for a long time. How often are patients discharged at short notice without *proper* consultation and preparation beforehand? How conscientious are all the professionals in checking that carers are able and equipped to receive patients back home and that all the services necessary are available and in place?

The Care Programme Approach details the importance of discharge planning. Section 117 of the Mental Health Act requires that all people detained under Section 3 or who have been in hospital longer than six months must have a pre-discharge planning meeting at which all arrangements are clarified and all those who will be involved in the aftercare of the patient have agreed to their part in the care plan. Nurses, and in particular community psychiatric nurses, have a crucial role as care coordinators. All these areas have implications for the practice of nurses for which they will be increasingly accountable.

Advocacy

The movement towards patient empowerment which is implicit in the Patient's Charter has consequences for all people working in the mental health field. Nurses have for some time regarded themselves as advocates for the patients in their care, but, as the Community Psychiatric Nurses' Association states in its document 'A call for action: the CPNA response to the 1993 Mental Health Nursing Review' (CPNA, 1993), 'mental health nurses are sadly lacking in skills to be good advocates for their clients and patients', and calls for an investment in time and money towards a higher quality of advocacy. Mental health nurses must first accept the need for proper advocacy services to be available, and welcome them on the wards and encourage access to them in the community, before they can truly consider themselves advocates for those in their care.

The term 'citizen advocacy' means that someone is acting and speaking for an individual or group, expressing what the individual or group wishes to be said, but who does not necessarily have to have been in a similar situation. Advocates should never interpolate their own interpretation or opinions. Their function is to represent what the other person wishes.

'Peer advocacy' entails someone who has experienced mental illness, an ex-user of mental health services, speaking for someone who is a current user of the services, or who is present to support that user when trying to achieve change or to express concern to those in authority.

The User Movement in Britain grew from the examples set in the Netherlands and the USA. 'Survivors Speak Out' and the National Advocacy Movement have grown and spread across the country with local groups developing from Nottingham to Brighton, from Cambridge to Cardiff. Some groups have been able to influence major decisions in the development and change of service provision. The challenge for the future is how widely and quickly this movement of user participation, or patient empowerment, grows in Great Britain, and how enthusiastically mental health services embrace the work of advocates for people with mental health problems.

COMMUNITY CARE ACT 1990

The Community Care Act 1990 has introduced legislation designed to ensure that the needs of the most vulnerable groups of society are met through a system of needs-led assessment. The Government has given social services departments the authority to allocate funds for packages of care that have been agreed in consultation with clients, their carers and professional workers to suit the needs of each individual. Mental health nurses have a significant role to play in assisting with the assessment process and in determining the best and most appropriate level and type of care for all people with mental health problems.

The Care Programme Approach charges mental health teams to consider in detail the needs of people with continuing severe mental illness and those particularly at risk of relapse or of harming themselves or others. Primary nurses in hospital and community psychiatric nurses in the community are seen as key personnel in ensuring the continuity of care for the most vulnerable people with mental health problems. Nurses will need to acquire new skills in following up these people in such a way as to encourage them to engage in care programmes that offer hope and meaning, leading to a better quality of life and helping both clients and carers to understand the illness and manage the behaviour that accompanies the illness.

Rather than introduce new legislation in the form of compulsory supervision orders, as recently suggested by the Royal College of Psychiatrists, which would give powers to community mental health workers to ensure people complied with the treatment prescribed to them, it would seem more appropriate for all people working with this small but very vulnerable group, who seem unable to accept their need for treatment or care, to learn better ways of managing care. Media attention on isolated incidents, such as that of the young man who climbed into the lion's cage, only serves to increase the public's negative image of mental illness. Part of the solution must be to improve society's attitude to mental health. What role can nurses play in achieving this change?

HOMELESSNESS AND THE MENTALLY ILL

Since the decision was made in the late 1970s, following the publication of the Government's White Paper *Better Services for the Mentally Ill* (Department of Health and Social Security, 1975), that the old Victorian psychiatric hospitals should close and that provision for people with mental health problems should be provided in more community-based facilities, the number of people 'living rough' has increased. Public concern has forced health authorities to examine their policies and to address the problems of the homeless population who also have mental illnesses.

This has raised awareness of the fact that people who have severe mental health problems, such as schizophrenia, chronic depression or manic–depressive psychosis, are often unable to sustain the standard of living or behaviour required of people living in the community. They frequently lose their housing for one reason or another and spend what money they do have on drink, drugs or cigarettes. Because of this chaotic lifestyle, mental health professionals who usually lead orderly lives around appointments, clinics, a regular working day, find this group of people difficult to follow up and treat once they have left hospital.

The Care Programme Approach, introduced by the Department of Health in 1989, and the Community Care Act 1990 which became fully operational in 1993, both attempt to address the problems of caring for people with severe mental health problems discharged into the community and to minimize the incidence of people becoming homeless in the first place. This is an area of psychiatric care that still is sadly neglected in many parts of the country and which nurses can do much to influence by their attitude to this group of people. Research has shown that this group do not always receive the attention to aftercare planning that is given to those that are housed.

In some districts, specialist teams of mental health workers, including doctors, nurses, psychologists, occupational therapists and social workers, are working specifically with the homeless, identifying those who have a history of mental illness, ensuring that they are registered with a GP, assisting them to find stable housing and some kind of meaningful activity, and ensuring that they receive the attention and psychiatric follow-up that they need to prevent further mental health breakdown. They liaise closely with GPs and in some areas named GPs are known to hold clinics for the homeless. Where this occurs there is a quicker response to the need for psychiatric assessment. Admission to hospital can often be avoided, problems dealt with, medication prescribed and given in a way that individuals find less threatening and which is more likely to result in compliance and consistency of care. However, as funding is increasingly tight, solutions like this suffer from being part of a local agenda. How can nurses represent and advocate for this disenfranchised group?

ETHNIC MINORITIES

As already mentioned in Chapter 2, the mental health needs of ethnic minority groups have not been truly understood by the mental health services in this country. More research needs to be carried out and greater attention given to the cultural heritage of people from other countries and races. Mental health nurses have much to contribute in this field, especially as many qualified nurses already practising can teach and educate their colleagues about the culture, the way of life and religious beliefs of the countries from which they come.

COURT DIVERSION SCHEMES

Society and governments have been concerned that too many people are sent to prison who have got themselves into trouble with the law, not because they are criminals but because they have a mental illness that has caused them to behave in an irresponsible way. Forensic psychiatric services have been developed alongside general psychiatry to address this problem. People are assessed by staff from the forensic psychiatry department and magistrates are advised as to the appropriate placement in a psychiatric hospital. This has caused psychiatric nurses some anxiety. It has been observed that more people admitted into acute psychiatric wards nowadays are extremely distressed and seriously disturbed. The nature of the work that nurses are required to cope with on the wards can be equated to intensive care work with its emphasis on 'constant, concentrated nursing input in an atmosphere that can be tense and volatile' (Thomas, 1993). It is essential that nurses have the right training and skills to care for these people. This may well mean that new and imaginative ways need to be developed that allow this group to preserve their dignity and respect and be supported to return to a more ordered life in the community.

RESEARCH

Throughout this book the authors have made reference to the importance of nursing practice being soundly based in research findings. Desmond Cormack (1991) states in the Preface to the second edition of *The Research Process in Nursing* that 'Not all nurses will carry out research work, although the potential for all professional nurses to do so exists. Many nurses will choose to remain consumers of the research undertaken by others. A thorough understanding of the research process . . .

however, is essential to both researchers and consumers of research. Thus, all professional nurses should acquire an understanding of the research process in nursing'.

Most training courses now include a module which at the very least introduces nurses to the ideas of research, familiarizing them with the concepts and principles of the research process. Nurses may be shown how to identify key areas of interest, particularly those areas where there may be a gap in knowledge or understanding. They are very likely to be shown how to conduct a literature search, how to review and evaluate that literature search so as to extract those texts that are most relevant to the topic concerned. Nurses undergoing post-registration training courses are encouraged to engage in a research project which, due to the restrictions of the time scale of the course, cannot be too ambitious. However, this does contribute to raising awareness of previous studies, of the steps involved in undertaking research and in developing an ability to analyse critically current knowledge and thinking. The next step is to learn how to apply the results of research to the actual practice of nursing, whether in hospital or in the community.

Nursing in mental health is crying out for good, rigorous research studies to establish good practice which is of greatest benefit in improving the way care is delivered to people with mental health problems. It is no longer acceptable for nurses to do things because they have always been so. Nurses should be questioning and examining what is the best practice, and then developing their practice based on objective and scientifically tested information.

Most regional health authorities have a research directorate which includes a research nurse who leads nursing research in that region, providing advice and support to those engaging in research. Some health authorities and trusts employ research nurses to fulfil a similar role within their organization. There are an increasing number of nursing research units attached to university departments where students are encouraged to question, to think, to read and to investigate. By embarking on research projects, which may be either of a quantitative or a qualitative nature, so the body of knowledge and new skills based on that knowlege can be developed. An example of this has been used in Chapter 9 where research into families with a member suffering from a schizophrenic illness revealed information relating relapse to high expressed emotion. This led to new ways of working with families to help them to understand the dynamics of the relationships between the different members of the family and to CPNs learning new skills in psychosocial intervention (Brooker, 1993).

MENTAL HEALTH NURSING REVIEW

Since the last review of mental health nursing in 1968 there have been considerable changes in mental health care, brought about by changes in the philosophy and expectations of society and therefore of governments. The emphasis of care has moved from being institution based to being community based. This has led to the development of community mental health nursing with its exposure of nurses to working with primary health care teams. Nurses reacted with enthusiasm to the role of promoting mental health awareness among their colleagues and the public in general, in an attempt to break down fear and stigma associated with mental illness. This has led to criticisms of community mental health services neglecting the needs of those with severe mental illness in favour of those with milder but disabling mental health disorders. Both the Royal College of Nursing (1993) and the Community Psychiatric Nurses' Association (1993), in their responses to the National Review of Mental Health Nursing, make mention of the need to respond to the mental health needs of *all* people, and the importance of keeping a balance between providing a service for those with severe and continuing mental health needs and preventing mental illness through the promotion of good mental health practices.

They both emphasize the importance of retaining the specialist nature of mental health nursing and deplore the trend of reducing the number of training places for mental health nursing in colleges of education and, more recently, the decision allowing colleges no longer to provide all four branches under the Project 2000 training programme. The four branch programmes are general nursing, mental health nursing, mental handicap nursing and child health nursing. It is sincerely hoped that the Review will resist vigorously any temptation to conform with the model of mental health nurse training that occurs in the majority of European Union countries. Issues of training, education, status of mental health nursing, the responsiveness of mental health nursing services to the needs of local communities, the ability of nurses to work in different settings and their ability to be clear about what is special about mental health nursing must all be stated and supported so that nurses can concentrate on caring for people with mental health problems in as effective and efficient a way as possible.

An element of care that all nurses and mental health services will need to accept as part of their normal day's work in future in order to demonstrate this effectiveness and efficiency is that of clinical audit. This may be either audit of nursing care based on agreed standards, or multidisciplinary audit of teams of mental health workers by which standards of care are set and delivery of care is measured to see whether those standards are being met. Audit tools are being devised and tested across the country and adopted by services keen to improve the quality of care that they are giving to people with mental health problems. Standards of care should be set based on the most recent and up-to-date research which shows the most effective outcomes in care that are acceptable to patients and carers alike. How well are nurses working in mental health undertaking research themselves? How aware are they of research that has been done and how well are they able to apply these findings to their own practice? These questions are posed for the nurses of the future to respond to in order to take mental health nursing forward into the twenty-first century.

IN CONCLUSION

Mental health nursing faces a crossroads. The primary focus of care has moved from hospital to the community. This raises implications for the training of nurses. Where should it take place? Are current trained nurses equipped to assist in the training of new students? Is Project 2000 with its common foundation course and the branch programme sufficient to train nurses to care for people with severe mental health problems? Are the skills which nurses are taught now the most useful in caring for people with mental health problems? Having acknowledged that many of those who still require to be cared for in hospitals need intensive care, how best can nurses meet their needs?

The Community Care Act and *The Health of the Nation*

give ample scope for nurses to respond to the mental health needs of the communities in which they work, in whatever setting. We are living at a time of great change in the delivery of mental health care. Nurses must make sure that they are at the forefront of new developments, influencing decisions, based on good practice that is proven through robust and rigorous research.

FURTHER READING

Refer to the journals and quality newspapers in order to keep up-to-date with policy changes and developments.

New books and manuals dealing with specific skills and issues are frequently being published and are advertised in the nursing press.

REFERENCES

Brooker C, Tarrier N, Barrowclough C *et al.* (1993) Skills for CPNs working with seriously mentally ill people: the outcome of a trial of psychosocial intervention, in Community Psychiatric Nursing. *A Research Perspective* 2: 46–70.

Cormack D (1991) *The Research Process in Nursing*, second edition. Oxford: Blackwell Scientific Publications.

CPNA (1993) A call for action: the CPNA response to the 1993 Mental Health Nursing Review. *Community Psychiatric Nursing Journal* 13(2): 32–38.

Department of Health (1989) *Caring for People—Community Care in the Next Decade and Beyond*. London: HMSO.

Department of Health (1990) *The NHS and Community Care Act 1990*. London: HMSO.

Department of Health (1991) *The Patient's Charter*. London: HMSO.

Department of Health (1992) *The Health of the Nation*. London: HMSO.

Department of Health (1993) *A Vision for the Future: The Nursing, Midwifery and Health Visiting Contribution to Health and Health Care*. London: HMSO.

Department of Health and Social Security (1975) *Better Services for the Mentally Ill*. Cmnd 6233. London: HMSO.

Gournay K (1992) Psychiatric nursing in the nineties. *Nursing Standard* **6**(36): 50–52.

Royal College of Nursing (1992) *The Health of the Nation: A Response from the Royal College of Nursing*. London: RCN.

Royal College of Nursing (1993) *Evidence to the National Review of Mental Health Nursing*. London: RCN.

Thomas B (1993) Nurses must adapt to changes in hospital psychiatric care. *British Journal of Nursing* **2**(14): 698–699.

APPENDICES

Appendix A
Classification and Description of Some Psychiatric Disorders

The classification of psychiatric disorders has been the subject of much debate and often controversy in psychiatry. An outline of one possible, though not ideal, system of classification is given in this appendix, together with a brief description of some of the features of the disorders classified. A textbook of psychiatry should be consulted for fuller details of various psychiatric disorders.

Psychiatric disorders may be classified initially into two very broad groupings. The distinction is made between those disorders in which the aetiology is known, for example the *organic* psychiatric disorders, having a demonstrable underlying—and in the acute form often curable—physical cause, and those disorders described as *functional*, whose aetiology is not yet proved and therefore cannot be primarily attributed to a physical cause.

ORGANIC PSYCHIATRIC DISORDERS

Organic psychiatric disorders may be divided broadly into acute and chronic states. The acute organic disorders include acute confusion; the chronic disorders are associated with intellectual impairment e.g. dementia—see Chapter 10.

The term organic psychoses (as distinct from the functional psychoses—see below) may be applied to certain of the organic (acute) psychiatric disorders with clinical features which include delusions and hallucinations (especially visual and tactile) due, as has been said above, to an underlying physical cause. They include such states as drug intoxication and also alcohol withdrawal (delirium tremens). The terms *delusion* and *hallucination* will be described below.

FUNCTIONAL PSYCHIATRIC DISORDERS

It is convenient to subdivide the functional psychiatric disorders into two broad categories: (a) the (functional) neuroses and (b) the functional psychoses.

The (Functional) Neuroses

The neuroses, or neurotic reactions (to stress, for example), are those disorders in which *anxiety* is a predominant feature.

Anxiety may be overt or it may be transferred to a feared object or situation (phobias—irrational fears); underlying anxiety may be kept at bay only if the person is allowed to perform a certain action (ritual—compulsive action) or a series of actions (as in obsessive–compulsive states).

Rarely, anxiety is 'converted' (at an unconscious level) to a 'physical' symptom—one which allows the individual to opt out of an anxiety-provoking situation (e.g. a woman who quarrels incessantly with her husband suddenly develops *aphonia*—loss of voice, not attributable to a physical cause, unlike aphasia or dysphasia—inability to speak or difficulty in speaking due to an underlying neurological deficit).

In neuroses the person's emotional experiences and behaviour are *quantitatively* rather than *qualitatively* different from normal (cf. functional psychoses below). For example it is normal to feel anxious before sitting an examination, but this anxiety is not usually excessive and subsides as the situation progresses and one concentrates on the task in hand. In a neurotic disorder, however, the anxiety is multiplied thousandfold in a variety of situations, and may even become so severe that it interferes markedly with the person's daily life (see also Chapter 11).

The Functional Psychoses

The functional psychoses are psychiatric disorders which are characterized by their severity; they produce markedly disordered and disturbed behaviour, which is *qualitatively* rather than *quantitatively* different from normal and cannot be understood (as in the neuroses—see above) as an extension of ordinary, everyday experience. Patients with a psychotic disorder frequently lack insight (recognition by the person that he is ill) into their illness (unlike those with a neurotic disorder) and are often out of touch with reality. Other features associated with the functional psychoses, and which also distinguish this group from the neuroses, include the presence of *delusions* and *hallucinations*. (These occur in the presence of clear consciousness and with no underlying physical cause; cf. organic psychoses above).

Delusions

A delusion is a false belief which, in the face of contrary evidence, is held with absolute conviction and is unmodifiable by appeals to reason or logic that would be acceptable to persons of the same religious or cultural background. (Age too must be considered—a child of four who firmly believes in Santa Claus cannot be described as suffering from a delusion.)

A delusion signifies a break with reality which justifies its description as a 'psychotic' symptom. However, the mere presence of a delusion is not diagnostic of any particular psychiatric disorder, though some types of delusion may be characteristic of certain conditions.

Delusions may be classified by (a) mode of origin, (b) content and (c) degree of systematization.

(a) Mode of origin. A distinction can be made between 'primary' and 'secondary' delusions. Primary delusions appear suddenly, fully developed and without warning, and are associated with schizophrenia. By contrast, secondary delusions may occur in most psychotic disorders, and arise as a response of the patient to other symptoms of the condition. Thus, for example, mood-congruent delusions of guilt and unworthiness may arise in the setting of the depressive state and delusions of persecution in schizophrenia when auditory hallucinations ('voices') are attributed to a hostile person or organization.

(b) Content. In terms of their content, several types of delusion are recognized. Delusions of grandeur may occur in mania and from time to time in schizophrenia. As the name implies, these are false beliefs concerning

the patient's status and power. Paranoid is the term used to describe all delusions of being affected in some harmful or persecutory way. These may occur not only in schizophrenia but also in affective disorders (see below) and organic psychoses (see above). It should be noted, however, that paranoid delusions *when associated with schizophrenia of late onset* (schizophrenia often occurs for the first time in late teens and early twenties) are typically well-systematized (see below) and usually accompanied by auditory hallucinations. But, importantly, in this type of schizophrenia there is preservation of the person's personality and he may be apparently normal in other respects. In severe depression the person experiencing paranoid delusions will commonly accept such 'persecution' as his just due, in keeping with his feeling of guilt and self-reproach. Delusions of reference are common in schizophrenia, but may also occur in affective illness, e.g. depression. The person believes that people, things and events refer to him in a special way. Thus people, even complete strangers in the street, look at him and he 'knows' they are talking about him, or items on television or in the newspaper are really referring to him. Somatic delusions are common in depression; a frequent complaint is blockage of the bowels. The person may insist his bowels have not moved for several weeks and that he ought to be transferred to a general hospital for urgent surgery. Somatic delusions may arise from unusual bodily sensations in schizophrenia. They are frequently bizarre; the patient believing, for example, that his appearance has completely changed and that he is turning into a woman. Nihilistic delusions may occur in psychotic depression. The individual believes that he is destroyed in part or totally, so that, for example, his inside has rotted away or he is already dead and in hell.

(c) Degree of systematization. The degree of logical relationship between delusions may vary. At one extreme, patients with a diagnosis of 'paranoid schizophrenia' may develop a system of delusions that is constructed in a logical manner and based on a single original false belief. Such delusions are said to be systematized. At the other extreme, delusions in acute organic psychoses (e.g. delirium tremens) are commonly short lived, changeable and unconnected with each other, i.e. unsystematized.

Hallucinations

A hallucination is a false *sensory* perception which arises on its own, in the absence of a corresponding external stimulus. All sensory modalities may be involved, so that in simple terms a hallucination can mean seeing, hearing, smelling, tasting or feeling something that is not there.

A hallucination should be distinguished from an *illusion*, another disorder of perception more commonly found in organic states. An illusion involves misinterpreting or mistaking something that *is* seen or heard for something else. Illusions are not uncommon in young children with pyrexia; they may 'see' the large sunflowers on the wallpaper as frightening spiders.

Visual hallucinations occur in organic psychoses—classically in alcohol withdrawal (delirium tremens)—and may take the form of grotesque monsters or animals of a terrifying nature. Visual hallucinations are less common than auditory (see below) in schizophrenia. They have been reported in manic states, the content in keeping with the patient's prevailing mood of elation, e.g. the person 'sees' a large box from which emerges a spray of multicoloured flowers of every conceivable variety and as they waft heavenward others appear from the box to take their place.

Auditory hallucinations occur most frequently in schizophrenia but are also found—though less commonly—in certain other psychiatric disorders of a psychotic nature. Auditory hallucinations may occur in severe (psychotic) depression and the content is then a reflection of the person's depressed mood (mood-congruent). The patient may hear voices saying that he is evil, lives a sinful life and does not deserve the food he is being offered or the nurse's attention. In schizophrenia two voices may give a running commentary on some of the patient's actions. Auditory hallucinations may be recognizable or not, distinct or muffled, abusive and often of a frightening nature. They may interfere totally with the person's ability to concentrate; a student may have to give up university because the almost constant chattering of 'voices' is causing him to fall behind in his work.

Olfactory hallucinations may occur in schizophrenia, a patient claiming, for example, that he can smell gas with which enemies are poisoning him. *Gustatory hallucinations* occur occasionally in schizophrenia. A patient may complain of a change in the taste of food which indicates to him that he is being poisoned.

Tactile hallucinations may be found in organic psychosis and in schizophrenia. Tactile hallucinations such as those felt in schizophrenia may lead to secondary delusional interpretation by the patient, e.g. that harmful laser beams are being directed at him.

Classification of Functional Psychoses

The functional psychoses may be divided into two broad categories: the affective disorders and schizophrenia.

The Affective Disorders

The term *'affect'* in psychiatry is used to describe feeling, emotion, mood. In the affective disorders the disturbance occurs in the sadness/happiness aspect of *mood*. Affective disorders therefore are psychiatric conditions in which the predominant feature is a relatively prolonged change of mood to a degree which seriously distrupts the patient's daily life. The patient's affect may be abnormally low as in a depressive illness or abnormally elated as in mania (or more commonly hypomania). Depression, which has been called 'the common cold of psychiatry', is much more likely to occur than mania. Someone who experiences episodes of depression but occasionally has also to be admitted to hospital because of elation and overactivity, is said to suffer from a *bipolar illness* (or disorder). The term manic-depressive psychosis is also applied to this disorder. On the other hand a person who experiences depressive episodes only may be given the diagnosis of *unipolar illness* (or recurrent depression). *Endogenous* depression (occurring 'out of the blue' without any external trigger) and *psychotic* depression (when delusions and/or auditory hallucinations are part of the clinical features) are also terms used in association with major depression. The nurse need not be unduly concerned, however, with the precise diagnosis; the nursing care of the severely depressed person is the same irrespective of the clinical terminology used by the psychiatrist.

Causes of depressive disorders. Some of the possible causes of depression have been discussed in Chapter 7.

Bipolar illness (manic-depressive psychosis) is believed to be associated with inherited factors.

Recently, researchers using biological techniques have been finding increasing evidence that a dominant gene constitutes a necessary cause of bipolar illness. This may be clarified in the near future by ongoing studies in molecular genetics (Baron & Rainer, 1988).

Main features of a major depressive episode. The depressed person often feels and looks sad. He has no energy, his movements and thoughts are slow (retardation), he stoops, or sits with his head bent low. He does not wish to converse and says as little as possible, slowly and in monosyllables. He is uninterested in his surroundings, has difficulty in concentrating and in making the simplest of decisions. He is morbidly preoccupied with thoughts of hopelessness and despair which may lead to thoughts of suicide. The patient considers himself to be wicked, feels that he has committed unforgivable sins and that he deserves to be punished. He may hear voices which accuse him or comment on his unworthiness. His pessimistic concern with his wickedness or his poverty may be expressed as delusions. He may say that he lacks feeling altogether or feels empty.

Somatic symptoms include loss of appetite with resultant weight loss, sometimes constipation, loss of libido, amenorrhoea in female patients and insomnia. The depressed person may complain of early morning wakening (known as late insomnia)—as early as 2 a.m. or 3 a.m.

Causes of mania. A genetic cause of mania (as manifested in bipolar illness: manic–depressive psychosis) has been considered above. Given that a person is genetically vulnerable to pathological elation and overactivity, there is still considerable interest in the external factors or triggers which may precipitate a manic episode. It is postulated, for example, that certain stressful life events may sometimes trigger an episode. (See Appendix D for a scale of life events. Each event listed has a so-called life change unit (LCU) value alongside it: the higher the LCU score, the greater the potential for stress.) One example of a stressful life event, childbirth, is occasionally associated with the onset of mania though, as is well known, depression is much more common.

Carney *et al*. (1988) claim that weather may have an influence on the prevalence of mania; sunshine and day length correlated signficantly with admission rates, suggesting a supersensitivity to light in people prone to mania. (This contrasts with those who suffer from SAD (seasonal affective disorder)—a lowering of mood which coincides with the *lack* of daylight during winter months.)

Main features of a manic episode (see also p. 148). In mania the patient is elated and feels on top of the world. Everything is wonderful in his eyes; he is full of self-confidence, makes plans for great actions and indulges in feverish acitivity. His speech is so rapid that it may be difficult to follow ('pressure of talk'). The patient's movements are large, often graceful. There is constant activity, but inability to concentrate on any particular task. The patient feels constrained and hemmed in and is hypersensitive to noise. He is highly distractible. Any stimulus, a spoken word, a movement or some sound, will set off a new train of thought, word or actions.

Speech does not follow the usual logic. The sound of words is the cue to association of ideas ('clang association'). Rhyming and punning are common. Content may also be delusional and in keeping with the person's elated mood. For a while the patient's elation is infectious. Often his fellow patients are at first amused by him; later his kind intentions are looked upon as interferences and he may become a target of general hostility (see p. 153). In turn, the patient easily becomes irritable and sometimes aggressive to those in the vicinity if he is in any way prevented from carrying out his intentions.

Hypomania. This is a state of excitement and overactivity less severe than mania and more commonly seen nowadays. Recognition of early warning signs by the individual (or close relatives) that all is not well and that prompt professional help is needed will frequently abort a severe manic episode.

Schizophrenia

Schizophrenia represents a group of psychotic disorders which take a wide variety of forms with certain characteristics in common but with considerable variation in other respects.

Classification of schizophrenia. The traditional division of schizophrenia by Emil Kraepelin (1855–1926) into four subgroups—*simple, hebephrenic, catatonic* and *paranoid*—is still included in the *International Classification of Diseases: Classification of Mental and Behavioural Disorders* (WHO, 1992). According to this classification *simple* is uncommon and difficult to diagnose and *catatonic* is now rarely seen in industrial countries. The fourth subgroup, *paranoid*, is said to be the commonest type seen in 'most parts of the world'.

A more recent classification of schizophrenia is between acute or Type I syndrome, and chronic (nonacute) or Type II. In Type I the person presents with *positive* symptoms such as disturbing hallucinations, delusions (often bizarre), thought disorder (see below) and social withdrawal. A Type II syndrome, sometimes known as a deficit state, is characterized by *negative* symptoms which include a reduction in normal responses to environmental stimuli, such as poverty of speech (alogia) and thought, loss of drive (avolition), emotional and social withdrawal, difficulty in establishing interpersonal relationships and lack of self-care skills. Overlap between Types I and II is not uncommon. For example, a patient with negative symptoms may show some of the florid positive symptoms should he feel pressurized when participating in an active rehabilitation programme for which he has been inadequately prepared.

Main features of a schizophrenia episode. Many of the features of schizophrenia have been considered above (see also delusions and hallucinations); only disturbance of thought and emotional responsiveness require further elucidation.

Disordered thought processes. The nature of the malfunctioning of the person's thought processes (mainly in Type I) seldom occurs in any other mental disorder. Disturbance of the *content* of thought (delusions) has already been described above, but disturbances of connection and possession of thought may also be present.

- *Connection*: Many people with schizophrenia have difficulty in putting their thoughts together in a comprehensible manner, giving rise to a failure on the listener's part to grasp precisely what it is the patient is trying to communicate. Disconnected thinking is found in 'knight's move'—changes of topic not logically linked in any way; *thought blocking* may also occur—the person suddenly stops his line of thought appears to forget completely what he is saying, then continues, sometimes on an unrelated theme.

- *Possession*: Disturbance of possession of thought (or *thought control*) in schizophrenia may be divided into:
  - *thought insertion*: the person complains of thoughts being put into his head by some other person or agency;
  - *thought withdrawal*: the person says that his thoughts are being taken out of his head;
  - *thought broadcasting*: the person feels that his thoughts are being made available to others and that they know what he is thinking.

Disturbance of emotional responsiveness. In so-called *blunting or flattening of affect* the person shows a lack of emotional response; his voice and facial appearance lack any expression of emotion. Sometimes his response is inappropriate—an outburst of giggling when a sad topic is being discussed (*incongruity of affect*). Both these disturbances may be seen in Type I and II syndromes.

FURTHER READING

Gournay K (1990) A return to the medical model? *Nursing Times* **86**(40): 46–47.

Ironbar O & Hooper A (1989) *Self-instruction in Mental Health Nursing.* London: Baillière Tindall.

Lyttle J (1986) *Mental Disorders: Its Care and Treatment.* London: Baillière Tindall, pp. 127–128.

Sims A (1988) *Symptoms in the Mind.* London: Baillière Tindall.

REFERENCES

Baron M & Rainer J (1988) Molecular genetics and human disease. *British Journal of Psychiatry* **152**: 741–753.

Carney PA, Fitzgerald CT & Monagnam CE (1988) Influence of climate on the prevalence of mania. *British Journal of Psychiatry* **152**: 820–824.

World Health Organisation (1992) *The ICD-10 Classification of Mental and Behavioural Disorders: Clinical Descriptions and Diagnostic Guidelines*. Geneva: WHO.

Appendix B
Notes on the Mental Health Act 1983 and the Mental Health (Scotland) Act 1984

HISTORICAL OVERVIEW

In the course of the last 100 years, legislation has been in existence to protect people who, by virtue of their mental disorder, are deemed to be vulnerable to abuse from members of the public and from unscrupulous members of staff of the institutions in which they are being cared for.

At the end of the nineteenth century, the Lunacy Acts and the Mental Deficiency Acts were primarily designed to prevent compulsory detention in an 'asylum' of anyone who was not a danger to others or to him/herself as well as suffering from a mental disorder. Apart from the many sections of these Acts which regulated admission to institutions, discharge from and care while in an institution, the Acts made provision for 'The Board of Control', a watchdog body with the duty to exercise protective functions on behalf of the mentally disordered.

The way the Lunacy Acts operated made it difficult, however, for people to obtain care and treatment unless they were in danger or a danger to others. In the 1930s, new legislation, the Mental Treatment Acts, made it possible to admit mentally disordered people, now referred to as 'patients', to institutions, renamed 'hospitals', on a voluntary basis. The protection against abuse which the Acts afforded applied also to voluntary patients.

To become a voluntary patient it was necessary to sign an application and patients had to give notice in writing of their intention to discharge themselves.

It was necessary to ensure that patients really understood what they were doing, and a medical officer had to ascertain that the patient was indeed 'volitional'. Many patients, though perfectly willing to be in hospital, were deemed not to be suitable for voluntary status because they were not regarded as volitional. Demented patients, confused patients, severely depressed patients or schizophrenic patients who were very withdrawn, and severely mentally handicapped people had to be admitted under 'certificate' for this reason.

In the 1950s a Royal Commission recommended changes in legislation and in 1959 in England and Wales, 1960 in Scotland and 1961 in Northern Ireland, new legislation—'The Mental Health Acts'—came into operation. The main principles on which the Acts were based were:

1 That patients suffering from mental disorder should as far as possible be treated, in or outside hospital, on the same basis as patients suffering from any other disorder. They should be able to enter any hospital capable of offering treatment. They should enter hospital or leave hospital with no more formality or restrictions than any other patients.
2 That, outside hospital, provisions should be made for treatment and care comparable to those offered to people suffering from other disorders.
3 That hospitals which offered psychiatric treatment should be free to refuse admission if they felt unable to help the patient or for any other reason, just as other hospitals are.
4 That the provisions made for the fairly small number

of patients who must be detained against their will should entail only a minimal amount of legal restriction.

5 In England and Wales, that special provisions for protection were no longer necessary.

In order to achieve these objectives, all previous legislation relating both to mental illness and what was formally known as mental deficiency was repealed. One Act replaced all former legislation and it covered disorders not formerly dealt with.

The term 'mental disorder' was used to cover all disorders dealt with under the Act. The definition in the Act of 'Mental Disorder' was: 'Mental illness, arrested or incomplete development, psychopathic disorder and any other disorder or disability of mind'. In Scotland the term 'psychopathic disorder' was not used.

There were four subdivisions of mental disorder recognized for the purposes of the compulsory provisions of the Act of 1959:

1 Mental illness
2 Severe subnormality
3 Subnormality
4 Psychopathic disorder

The Scottish Act did not define the categories. The term 'mental disorder' meant 'mental illness and mental defect. The latter term remained in use.

Admission without compulsion. Patients in all four of these categories could be admitted to any hospital without compulsion or application. It was not necessary that the patient should be capable of expressing a wish to be admitted. As long as he was not actively unwilling to enter hospital his admission could be informal.

Compulsory admission. In England and Wales and in Northern Ireland, for those patients who had to be admitted against their will, only the signatures of two specifically designated doctors were necessary. In Scotland, only emergency admissions were possible on the authority of medical officers. Within seven days an application to the Sheriff had to be made to obtain his authority for further compulsory detention.

In England and Wales and in Northern Ireland, no watchdog organization was appointed. When the Board of Control was dissolved in Scotland, the Mental Welfare Commission was appointed with the general brief of exercising protective functions. It had less power, however, than its predecessor, the Board of Control.

By the end of the 1970s it had become clear that the legislation of the 1960s had provided insufficient safeguards for patients. Following a review, a new Mental Health Act was passed in 1983 and a new Mental Health (Scotland) Act in 1984.

THE MENTAL HEALTH ACT 1983

Application of the Act

The Act concerns 'the reception, care and treatment of mentally disordered patients, the management of their property and other related matters'. The definition of mental disorder is a mental illness, arrested or incomplete development of mind, psychopathic disorder or any other disorder or disability of mind. For most purposes of the Act it is enough for a patient to be suffering from one of the four specific categories of mental disorder set out in the Act:

1 Mental illness
2 Mental impairment: severe
3 Mental impairment: significant
4 Psychopathic disorder

It is important to note that no person shall be treated as suffering from mental disorder by reason of promiscuity or other immoral conduct, sexual deviancy, or dependence on alcohol or drugs.

The Scottish Act does not define the categories. The words mental subnormality and mental deficiency cease to have effect.

Admission without Compulsion

Informal admission should be the normal mode of admission to hospital whenever a patient is willing to be admitted and be treated without the use of compulsory powers. It is not necessary that the patient should be capable of expressing a wish to be admitted. As long as he is not actively unwilling to enter hospital the admission can be informal. The majority of patients enter hospital as informal admissions.

Compulsory Admission: England and Wales

Some patients suffering from mental disorder may have to be compulsorily admitted to and detained in hospital or received into guardianship. There are a number of different powers under which a patient may be compulsorily detained in hospital:

Admission for Assessment in Cases of Emergency (Section 4)

An application may be made by an approved social worker or by the nearest relative of the patient in exceptional circumstances. The applicant must state that it is of urgent necessity that the patient should be admitted and detained for assessment, and that compliance with the normal procedures would involve undesirable delay. Only one medical recommendation is required, but the practitioner concerned must have seen the patient within the previous 24 hours. The application is effective for 72 hours.

Admission for Assessment (Section 2)

Admission to and detention in hospital for assessment may be authorized where a patient is (a) suffering from mental disorder of a nature or degree which warrants the detention of the patient in hospital for assessment (or for assessment followed by medical treatment) for at least a limited period and (b) he ought to be so detained in the interests of his health or safety, or with a view to the protection of others. Detention is for up to 28 days. An application for admission must be made by either the patient's nearest relative or an approved social worker. An application for admission must be accompanied by written recommendations from two medical practitioners, one of whom must be approved as having special experience in the diagnosis and treatment of mental disorder.

Admission for Treatment (Section 3)

The grounds for admission for treatment are first that the patient is suffering from one or more of the four forms of mental disorder as previously described. Secondly, the mental disorder must be of a nature or degree which makes it appropriate for the patient to receive medical treatment in hospital. Thirdly, for a patient suffering from psychopathic disorder or mental impairment there is an additional condition that medical treatment is likely to alleviate or prevent a deterioration in the patient's condition. Treatment need not be expected to cure the patient's disorder: medical treatment should enable the patient to cope more satisfactorily with his disorder or it should stop his condition from becoming worse. Fourthly, it must be necessary for the health or safety of the patient or for the protection of others that he should receive this treatment and it cannot be provided unless he is detained. Application for admission for treatment must be made by either an approved social worker or the patient's nearest relative. The person who is to be regarded as nearest relative is defined in the Act. This must be accompanied by written recommendations from two medical practitioners, one of whom must be approved as having special experience in diagnosis and treatment of mental disorder. Detention for treatment is for a maximum period of six months unless the order is renewed.

Patients Already in Hospital (Section 5(2))

A patient already receiving inpatient treatment may be compulsorily detained for up to 72 hours if the doctor in charge of his treatment reports that an application for admission ought to be made.

Nurses' Holding Power (Section 5(4))

An important innovation of this Act is the nurses' holding power. If the doctor is not obtainable, a first level nurse trained in nursing people suffering from mental illness may detain an informal patient on behalf of the managers for a period of up to six hours while a doctor is found. It must appear to the nurse that (a) the patient is suffering from mental disorder to such a degree that it is necessary for his health or safety, or for the protection of others, for him to be immediately restrained from leaving hospital and (b) it is not practicable to secure the immediate attendance of a doctor for the purpose of furnishing a report. The nurse must record these facts in writing.

Mental Health Review Tribunal (MHRT)

Patients who feel they are wrongfully detained may apply to a Mental Health Review Tribunal to have their case considered. The tribunal has the power to discharge a patient from hospital. Patients admitted for assessment may apply within the first 14 days of detention. Patients admitted for treatment may apply within the first six months of detention, and again within six months if the detention order is renewed. A Mental Health Act Commission ensures that hospitals have adopted and are following proper procedures for using the powers of detention. The Commission also assists in staff guidance on good practice, which is included in a Code of Practice. The Mental Health Act Commission is a multidisciplinary and independent group set up by the 1983 Act. It is concerned with the welfare and protection of all detained patients.

Patients' Information

The hospital managers must provide certain information to detained patients and their nearest relatives. This is to ensure that the detained patient understands the nature of his detention and his right to apply to a Mental Health Review Tribunal. They must also inform the person with whom the patient has last been living.

Consent to Treatment

Compulsory detention does not mean that the patient may be automatically compelled to accept treatment. There are safeguards to ensure that either a second opinion or consent to treatment or both are obtained in the case of certain forms of treatment.

*Treatment Requiring Consent **and** a Second Opinion (Section 57)*

This section of the Act applies to the following forms of treatment where outcome is irreversible.

1 Psychosurgery—any surgical operation for destroying brain tissues or the function of the brain.
2 Surgical implantation of hormones. The Mental Health Act Commission must be notified to consider the validity of the patient's consent. They will jointly issue a certificate but, before doing so, the medical member will consult with a nurse and one other professional who have been concerned with the patient's treatment.

*Treatment Requiring Consent **or** a Second Opinion (Section 58)*

This section of the Act applies to the following forms of treatment.

1 The administration of medicine if three months or more have elapsed since medicine was first administered during that period of detention.
2 Electroconvulsive therapy.

If the patient does not consent to a treatment, the Mental Health Act Commission must be consulted for a second opinion. In addition, the medical member will consult with a nurse and one other professional and the responsible medical officer before giving a second opinion.

Urgent Treatment (Section 62)

Special conditions are set out for treating patients in an emergency but they exclude those treatments mentioned above. Such treatments will be necessary to save the patient's life, to prevent serious deterioration of his condition, to alleviate serious suffering by the patient or to prevent the patient from behaving violently or being a danger to himself or to others. In cases where treatment is not immediately necessary or it is proposed to continue treatment after the initial urgent administration, it will be necessary to contact the Mental Health Act Commission.

Withdrawing Consent (Section 60)

If a patient withdraws his consent to any treatment, the treatment must not be given or must cease to be given immediately.

Powers of the Courts and the Home Secretary

In certain circumstances patients may be admitted to and detained in hospital on the order of a court, or may be transferred to hospital from penal institutions on the direction of the Home Secretary. The courts also have the powers: to remand to hospital for a medical report: to remand to hospital for treatment; and to obtain interim hospital orders.

Patients' property may be protected by the 'Court of Protection'.

APPLICATION OF THE MENTAL HEALTH (SCOTLAND) ACT 1984

Unlike the Mental Health Act Commission in England and Wales, *The Mental Welfare Commission* in Scotland is not new. Under the 1984 Act it has increased duties and increased power. It is concerned with exercising 'protective function in respect of mentally disordered persons who may be incapable of adequately protecting their persons or their interests', whether they are compulsorily detained or not, and wherever they are, whether in hospital or in the community. (The Mental Health Act Commission in England and Wales is concerned only with detained patients.)

In Scotland there is no Mental Health Review Tribunal. Detained patients may appeal for discharge either to the Sheriff or to the Mental Welfare Commission, which has the power to order the discharge of a patient against medical advice.

The Mental Welfare Commission has the duty to bring

to the attention of the managers any matter which they consider appropriate to secure the welfare of any patient by:

- preventing ill treatment;
- remedying any deficiency in care or treatment;
- preventing or redressing loss or damage to his property.

Curator bonis

The Mental Welfare Commission has the power to petition for the appointment of a *curator bonis* to administer a patient's property and affairs.

The duties of the Mental Welfare Commission to visit, interview and examine patients who are compulsorily detained and to visit patients on leave of absence, and the power to hold enquiries and require persons to give evidence, are laid down in the Act.

Compulsory Detention of Patients

Provisions for Emergency Admission (Section 24) are similar to those in England and Wales. The term 'short-term detention' is used for detention up to 28 days (Section 26) and 'long-term detention' for a period of detention beyond that (Section 18). Short- and long-term detention must be authorized by the Sheriff.

Nurses have the power to detain a patient for only two hours (Section 25(2)).

The Mental Welfare Commission is informed at specified intervals of the movements in and out of hospital, of renewal of authority to detain a patient and of matters concerning guardianship.

Safeguards concerning consent to treatment are similar to those which apply in England and Wales (Sections 97 and 98).

Patients may be detained in hospital on the order of a court under the Criminal Procedure (Scotland) Act 1975. The Secretary of State is empowered to make an order restricting discharge.

GUARDIANSHIP

This form of legal control can be exercised over persons aged 16 years and over and is used as an alternative to hospital detention. Procedures and safeguards are similar to those in Section 18.

A social worker will be responsible for either choosing who the guardian will be or accepting as suitable the person nominated by the nearest relative.

If the patient resides in local authority accommodation the nominated guardian will then be chosen by the local authority. The nominated guardian who will usually be living with the patient must exercise effective control over him. The guardian's powers over the patient include:

- specifying his place of residence;
- ensuring his attendance for treatment, occupation, education or training;
- ensuring that access to the patient is given to specific people, e.g. medical practitioner or Mental Health Officer.

The guardian, however, has no power over the patient's property. Guardianship ceases if the patient remains absent without leave for 28 days.

Appendix C
Drugs and Pharmacology in Psychiatry

In the past four decades the introduction of effective drugs has dramatically changed the practice of psychiatry and psychiatric nursing. These drugs have made a significant contribution to the move from institutional to community care. Chlorpromazine (Largactil), the first effective drug for schizophrenia, appeared in the early 1950s followed shortly afterwards by effective antidepressant medication.

ADMINISTRATION OF MEDICATION: THE NURSE'S ROLE

In earlier chapters the nurse's role in administering and monitoring the effects of medication and in encouraging patient compliance has been emphasized, as have the appropriate nursing interventions when side-effects may be a problem.

Fortunately not all patients develop adverse reactions to the drugs used in psychiatry: responses cannot be predicted and the dose, type of drug, route of administration and patient's age are all variables to be taken into account.

It is important, however, that prompt attention is drawn to the appearance of any unwanted effects if and when they do occur; certain observations should be charted before a patient commences drug therapy so that a baseline reading is available and deviations identified at an early stage. Examples might include the patient's temperature, blood pressure and weight. The rationale for specific nursing observations—particularly during early stages of the administration of medication—is given later after the relevant drugs have been outlined. In this appendix only a few of the more commonly used drugs will be described, under the following headings:

1 Drugs used for the person who is depressed
2 Drugs used for the person who is elated and overactive
3 Drugs used for the person who is experiencing hallucinations and disordered thinking

DRUGS USED FOR THE PERSON WHO IS DEPRESSED

In some types of clinical depression there would appear to be a *decrease* in the availability of certain chemical neurotransmitters in the brain, e.g. the monoamine serotonin (or 5-hydroxytryptamine (5-HT)—the so-called monamine theory of depression. Thus it is widely held that the therapeutic effects of antidepressant drug therapy rest on their action in *increasing* the availability of the above transmitter at the synaptic cleft of central (nervous) receptor sites in the brain. Theoretically this increase could be achieved by a number of different pharmacological mechanisms but only two of the most effective in practice will be considered here: administration of drugs which

- inhibit monoamine reuptake;
- inhibit the action of the enzyme, monoamine oxidase.

Monoamine Reuptake Inhibiting Drugs (MARI)

This category of drugs, as the name suggests, exercises an antidepressant action by, in all probability, blocking (preventing) the normal reuptake of monoamines by the pre-synaptic neuron, thus increasing, the availability of these substances at the synaptic cleft.

Drugs in this group include the *tricyclics* (or 'classical' antidepressants) first introduced in the second half of the 1950s and the *standard* against which all later antidepressants' efficiency is measured. *Imipramine* (Tofranil), the first of them, was followed by *amitriptyline* (Tryptizol—more sedating than imipramine and therefore useful should agitation, anxiety and sleep disturbance coexist with the low mood). Tricyclic antidepressants, especially amitriptyline, may adversely affect the heart and for patients with heartblock or arrhythmias one of the later ('second generation') antidepressants, e.g. mianserin (Bolvidon), may be used. Mianserin also has useful sedative properties but a number of reports of leucopenia (reduced white blood count) have been documented with its use and regular white blood counts are advised during the first three months of treatment. Weight gain and a risk of precipitating epileptiform seizures in susceptible individuals should also be noted with tricyclic drugs. Another disadvantage with these early antidepressants—one which has not yet been fully overcome—is the relatively slow onset of any therapeutic effect. The nurse must be aware of this timelag; it could be as long as 14 to 21 days before the person's mood shows any appreciable improvement. As a result of this it could be that a severely depressed and potentially suicidal patient, hitherto retarded in movements, acquires the necessary energy and drive after some days on antidepressant therapy to carry out his intention to commit suicide—his mood being still very low.

In the late 1980s new antidepressants, *fluvoxamine* (Faverin) and fluoxetine (Prozac) were introduced which *selectively* block the reuptake of serotonin. Fewer major side-effects have been reported so far with their use, but they are contraindicated for pregnant women and mothers who are breast-feeding, in epileptic patients and in those who are underweight. The most frequently recorded unwanted effects with both these drugs are gastrointestinal symptoms such as nausea and vomiting—occasionally so severe as to warrant the drugs being discontinued (Kay & Bailie, 1990). Two further *selective* (or specific) *serotonin reuptake inhibitors* (SSRIs) have appeared in recent years—paroxetine (Seroxat) and sertraline (Lustral)—but their efficacy over those already established has still to be proved.

Monoamine Oxidase Inhibitors (MAOIs)

One of the actions of the enzyme *monoamine oxidase* is thought to be associated with a degree of metabolic degradation (breakdown) of serotonin and thus its inactivation by MAOI drugs is followed by a therapeutic increase in the concentration of this amine at the synaptic cleft. Phenelzine (Nardil) is the most commonly used of this group of drugs, and while not so effective as the tricyclics in severe depression, it has a valuable role in the treatment of people with atypical depressive reactions, e.g. those who in addition to being depressed may show other clinical features: anxiety, lethargy and an increase in both appetite and sleep. Occasionally patients who do not respond to any of the other antidepressants may show a favourable reaction to one of the MAOIs.

Unwanted Effects of Monoamine Oxidase Inhibitors

1   *Liver damage*. This group of antidepressants may cause liver damage (idiosyncratic hepatotoxicity).

2   *Hypertensive crises* (*'cheese effect'*). One of the substances implicated in this serious, and potentially fatal, reaction is tyramine—a potent hypertensive agent found as a naturally occurring amine in the diet. Normally, most of this dietary tyramine, once ingested, is metabolized immediately by the monoamines in the intestinal mucosa and the liver. If a person is taking a MAOI, however, there is a reduction in the level of these intestinal and hepatic monoamines; dietary tyramine is therefore not handled as it should be, but is absorbed intact and enters the bloodstream causing prolonged release of noradrenaline (NA). The pressor effects evoked by NA may result in a sudden steep rise in the patient's blood pressure.

Cheese, containing as it does a high level of tyramine, was the foodstuff originally isolated as causing this chain reaction and has given it the name the 'cheese reaction' or 'cheese effect'.

Anyone taking a MAOI must always carry a special card to remind him of the other substances, as well as cheese, he must avoid. Included in the list are Marmite, Bovril and other yeast and meat extracts, broad bean pods (commonly eaten in some cultures), pickled herrings and some animal livers. Alcoholic drinks are best avoided; Chianti wine, for example, may contain up to 0.25 mg of tyramine per bottle. Nor are alcohol-free drinks safe; Murray *et al.* (1988) report that a 48-year-old man taking a MAOI for a depressive episode suffered a cerebrovascular accident 15 minutes after drinking only 250 ml of alcohol-free beer.

Everyday cough and cold 'cures' may contain sympathomimetic amines (substances which mimic the adrenergic effect (i.e. of the NA- or adrenaline-releasing neurons at the synapse) of the sympathetic nervous system). If taken unwittingly by a person receiving MAOIs such remedies may precipitate a hypertensive crisis (see below).

Nursing staff must know of these restrictions and ensure that the patient fully understands why it is necessary to comply with them and to carry a card on discharge from hospital.

Signs and symptoms of a hypertensive crisis. The patient affected may initially complain of a headache and this must be reported immediately by the nurse. Blood pressure increases of over 50 mmHg systolic and 30 mmHg diastolic have been recorded. The headache may worsen, becoming very severe, and is accompanied by palpitations, sweating, flushing, nausea and vomiting, or neck rigidity and photophobia. This crisis is treated with an adrenergic receptor blocking drug (a drug which has vasodilator properties; by preventing (blocking) further release of NA the blood pressure is lowered), such as phentolamine, 5–10 mg given by intravenous injection.

Drug Interactions with Monoamine Oxidase Inhibitors

Pethidine and certain other narcotic compounds must not be given to patients receiving MAOIs; serious, and occasionally fatal, toxic reactions have been reported.

If the prescription of a patient who is receiving a tricyclic antidepressant drug has to be changed to a MAOI, or vice versa, it is recommended that a two-week drug-free period be allowed before the new drug is commenced.

Theoretically, the MAOI might be expected to complement the action of the tricyclic drug, but in fact serious
reactions have been described when a combination has
been used.

Second-generation Monoamine Oxidase Inhibitors

A new drug, moclobemide, has been called the 'gentle
MAOI' by Priest (1989) because its mild and transient
pressor effects necessitate fewer dietary restrictions.
Should this drug prove to be as effective as other MAOIs
it may improve patient compliance—an understandable
problem with the older monoamine oxidase inhibitors.

General Unwanted Effects of Antidepressants

In addition to the specific unwanted reactions outlined
above, there are also a number of general side-effects,
occurring especially in the early stages of drug therapy,
which are common to most, if not all, antidepressant
drugs. The atropine-like (autonomic: parasympathic
blockade) action of these compounds gives rise to
dryness of the mouth, difficulty in visual accommodation
and constipation. Other unwanted effects are drowsiness, dizziness, tremor, unsteadiness of gait, postural
hypotension and difficulty with micturition.

Long-term Administration of Antidepressant Drugs

As with any drug, each patient varies in his or her
response to an antidepressant compound. Quite a few
different drugs may have to be tried in succession before

a favourable outcome is eventually reached. Should the patient suffer from recurrent depression, the psychiatrist may decide, on the patient's recovery from his latest admission, to continue with the successful drug for some considerable length of time—as long perhaps as five years with certain patients—after discharge from hospital.

Prophylaxis of Recurrent Depression

Lithium

Since the introduction of lithium salts in 1949 as a preparation of value in mania, hundreds of reports have been published covering all aspects of lithium therapy. Today, lithium enjoys an established reputation as a useful drug in reducing the recurrence rate of bipolar illness (see Appendix A).

Its mode of action is unclear but it is thought to produce a marked enhancement of the function of certain brain amines (e.g. serotonin) (Cowan, 1988). Claims have been made for the use of lithium in the *treatment* of certain types of depression but current practice does not support its use in preference to the other antidepressant drugs on the market.

Physical preparation of the patient. Before embarking on a course of lithium therapy the patient has an assessment of his renal and thyroid function; the principal route of the elimination of lithium from the body is by the kidneys and the thyroid gland has been known to be affected by lithium preparations.

Lithium is marketed as lithium carbonate, either as the preparation Camcolit, or as a slower release tablet, e.g. Liskonum.

Monitoring plasma levels of lithium. Therapeutic and toxic levels of lithium (Li^+) are close to one another and an appropriate plasma lithium level must be calculated for each patient. Patients have blood samples taken weekly during the first few weeks of treatment; many authorities recommend that the plasma concentration range should be between 0.4 and 0.8 mmol Li^+/litre. However, Silverstone and Turner (1988) suggest that monitoring intra-erythrocyte lithium concentration may be more effective in reducing the relapse rate of patients with recurrent depression. At least 12 hours must have elapsed between the ingestion of the last dose of lithium and the blood sample being taken from the patient. The nurse must know of this interval and make sure that the patient's medication is stopped at the appropriate time.

Once the acceptable dose of lithium has been established for the individual patient, the interval between serum estimations may be increased gradually, provided the patient remains well and shows no evidence of untoward reactions to the drug. The age of the patient should also be considered. Elderly people receiving lithium require more frequent monitoring because of the inherent reduction in renal functioning as a person grows older. Thyroid function tests are also carried out at regular intervals.

Unwanted effects of lithium. Pregnancy is a contraindication to the use of lithium. Lithium may cause malformation of the foetus if given during the first trimester. A woman is advised not to breast-feed if lithium has been prescribed for her. The drug passes into the breast milk causing adverse effects such as hypotonia and hypothermia in the baby. Alternatively, the mother may not take the lithium during the breast-feeding period, but this may not be advisable because someone prone to recurrent depressive episodes is especially vulnerable in the puerperium.

In view of the relatively narrow therapeutic range for lithium, it is important for the nurse and the patient to be aware of the signs and symptoms of impending toxicity. Before discharge the patient is given written information relating to side-effects, and because toxicity is potentially disorientating, members of the patient's immediate family should know how to recognize warning signs (see below).

It is useful to distinguish between (a) side-effects which are relatively common initially; some may persist beyond the first phase of treatment, and are upsetting for the patient, but nevertheless harmless; (b) later side-effects; and (c) prodromes of lithium intoxication.

Initial side-effects. Feelings of anorexia, nausea or a metallic taste in the mouth are not unusual. The last of those symptoms may be minimized if tablets are given during or after meals.

The patient may complain of dizziness and also a fine tremor of the hands; loose stools are often reported in the early stages of treatment. Other patients may find constipation, a dry mouth and thirst troublesome side-effects. Skin eruptions and an exacerbation of existing skin conditions have been reported.

Later side-effects. Weight gain may be noted and oedema may be present. Hypothyroidism has been known to develop and is treated with supplements of thyroxine. Persistent polyuria and polydipsia (known as reversible nephrogenic diabetes insipidus) may interfere with the patient's sleep. The night nurse may be the first person to report this side-effect if the patient is still in hospital.

Chronic renal damage has been reported as a long-term reaction to lithium. It is claimed that this has been due in the past to high levels of lithium and should not now occur provided toxicity is avoided.

Patients receiving lithium should be advised to avoid situations which give rise to prolonged sweating. The salt lost is replaced in the cells by lithium, with a consequent reduction in lithium clearance. This in turn gives rise to high blood levels of lithium and a risk of toxicity. A bout of food poisoning, which also causes electrolyte imbalance, could have serious consequences and medical advice should be sought.

Prodromes of lithium intoxication. Warning signs of impending toxicity are associated with symptoms of excessive thirst, frank vomiting and/or diarrhoea. Medical help should be sought immediately. Neurological signs include a coarse tremor, slurred speech, sleepiness, sluggishness, ataxia and mental confusion. The drug is withdrawn and the plasma level is measured as a matter of urgency. If prompt action is not taken in this medical emergency, the patient's condition will deteriorate rapidly. Sodium depletion is again a potential danger and saline may be infused intravenously for swift replacement, especially if the patient is vomiting. Patients with severe lithium poisoning may require haemodialysis.

Drug interactions with lithium. Increased sodium intake, in one form or another, can lead to increased lithium clearance with a resultant drop in serum levels (i.e. the opposite effect of sodium loss). Other compounds known to interfere with lithium clearance are diuretics and some anti-obesity drugs. They may cause lithium levels to rise. Lithium may potentiate the action of muscle relaxants; a note of the patient's medication is passed to the anaesthetist if and when the patient requires to have general anaesthesia.

Carbamazepine

The anticonvulsant drug, carbamazepine (Tegretol) may be used in psychiatry to prevent recurrent bipolar illness. It may be given alone or in combination with lithium. Carbamazine's mode of action may be due to its effect on the entry of sodium to the post-synaptic membrane. Side-effects associated with carbamazine include ataxia, gastrointestinal disturbances and drowsiness.

DRUGS USED IN THE TREATMENT OF THE PERSON WHO IS ELATED AND OVERACTIVE

Antipsychotic Drugs

The antipsychotic drugs, or neuroleptics, discussed in detail in the next part of this appendix, are frequently used in the treatment of the elated and overactive person; one which is particularly useful is haloperidol (Haldol) (a butyrophenone). The unwanted effects of haloperidol are similar to those found in patients receiving many of the other neuroleptics and they are also discussed later.

Lithium

Lithium (for details see above) may be used with therapeutic effect during a hypomanic episode but it can take up to a week before any improvement is noted and for this reason the quicker-acting haloperidol may be given first, followed later by lithium, as soon as the person has improved sufficiently to allow the initial drug to be reduced gradually as the lithium begins to take effect.

Prophylaxis of Recurrent Mania

Drugs used to reduce the risk of recurrence of a manic episode are the same as those used to prevent a recurrence of a depressive illness, i.e. lithium and carbamazepine.

DRUGS USED FOR THE PERSON WHO IS EXPERIENCING HALLUCINATIONS AND DISORDERED THINKING

Neuroleptic (or antipsychotic) drugs—formerly known as major tranquillizers—exert a therapeutic action on psychotic symptoms such as hallucinations and disordered thinking. It is convenient to classify neuroleptics according to the chemical 'family' they belong to and two examples will be briefly considered.

Phenothiazines

The first of the neuroleptics, *chlorpromazine* (Largactil), the standard phenothiazine, was first introduced in the early 1950s. This drug has a pronounced calmative effect on acutely disturbed patients when given by intramuscular injection.

Other examples of phenothiazines are:

- *Fluphenazine decanoate* (Modecate), a long-acting (depot) phenothiazine given by deep intramuscular injection. It is particularly valuable for the person in the community who fails to appreciate the need to continue with oral medication on a daily basis.
- *Thioridazine* (Melleril), a commonly used phenothiazine. It has fewer side-effects (see below) than chlorpromazine and is valuable in the treatment of the elderly person.

Thioxanthenes

The best known of this group are the long-acting injectable compounds *flupenthixol decanoate* (Depixol) and *zuclopenthixol decanoate* (Clopixol), chemically related to the phenothiazines and with similar therapeutic properties.

New Neuroleptics

Two new neuroleptics, clozapine (Clozaril) and risperidone (Risperdal) have been introduced into the UK in recent years. The first, clozapine (a dibenzodiazepine), is said by Launer (1992) to have a unique effect in severe schizophrenia, especially on negative symptoms previously drug-resistant, and to have fewer extrapyramidal effects than some of the earlier compounds. (Extrapyramidal is a clinical rather than an anatomical term. The extrapyramidal system roughly comprises all parts of the central nervous system concerned with the regulation of motor function (but excluding the pyramidal tracts, i.e. the motor tracts connecting the cortex and spinal cord).) Clozapine can only be used if the patient's white blood count is carefully monitored to detect leucopenia (lowering of white blood cells). Risperidone (a benzisoxazole) is also claimed to be beneficial in reducing the negative symptoms of schizophrenia. As with clozapine, risperidone is said to have a good side-effect profile (Cookson, 1993).

Unwanted Effects of Neuroleptic Medication

The extrapyramidal effects of neuroleptic medication will be looked at first—and in some detail—because of the distressing effect they can have on the well-being of the person with a schizophrenic disorder; other examples of side-effects associated with such drugs have been selected for their implications for nursing practice.

Extrapyramidal Symptoms (Disturbance of Motor Activity)

The extrapyramidal side-effects of neuroleptic drugs are best understood in terms of the biochemical approach to the study of the causes of schizophrenia—the so-called 'dopamine hypothesis'. (Dopamine, however, is only one of the many chemical neurotransmitters in the brain to have been identified in the past as an important neurotransmitter in the aetiology of schizophrenic disorders.) The dopamine theory, which lays claim to a hyperactivity or hyperreactivity of dopamine at the synapse, is not substantiated by unequivocal evidence: Reynolds (1989), however, suggests that this increased dopamine function might be secondary to a neuronal abnormality elsewhere in the brain. In any event the neurotransmitter dysfunctioning is 'corrected' by the administration of antipsychotic drugs whose mode of action is to *block dopamine receptors* on the post-synaptic cell membrane.

The unwanted (extrapyramidal) effects of neuroleptic drugs are the result of this dopamine blockade on post-synaptic cells in the corpus striatum (part of the extrapyramidal system—as the name of this group of side-effects suggests). It creates a *functional deficiency of dopamine*, the effects of which may be seen in a variety of disorders of motor activity because the corpus striatum is involved in regulating involuntary movement and muscle tone.

However, it is postulated that the *therapeutic* action of antipsychotic medication rests on essentially the same cellular mechanism, but their beneficial antidopaminergic activity is concentrated mainly in the *limbic system* in the brain. The limbic system is associated, in part, with a person's emotional behaviour.

These disorders of motor activity (i.e. the extrapyramidal side-effects due to dopamine depletion) may be considered under four headings: (a) acute dystonic reactions; (b) parkinsonian syndrome (drug-induced parkinsonism); (c) akathisia; and (d) tardive dyskinesia.

In the first *three* of these groups, symptoms diminish if the dose of the offending drug is reduced or the drug discontinued. If it is not advisable to take either of these steps, some of the symptoms may be counteracted by the oral administration of an antiparkinsonian agent, e.g. benzhexol (Artane) or procyclidine (Kemadrin). These drugs must be used with caution, however; problems include addiction to their mood-elevating properties and toxic confusional states.

The *fourth* group, tardive dyskinesia, is of particular concern because discontinuation of the drug has been known to worsen the symptoms. Attempts to find an effective treatment for this reaction are the subject of much current research.

The butyrophenones (see p. 341) and the depot preparations are especially liable to give rise to extrapyramidal side-effects, though it has been suggested recently that zuclopenthixol decanoate (Clopixol) may have a lower tendency to do so than the other injectable compounds.

(a) *Acute dystonic reactions*. The nurse's role in the early recognition of this distressing condition is vital. It appears early in treatment and is commoner in the younger male patient. It should not be mistaken for bizarre posturing sometimes seen in schizophrenia. Involuntary contraction of the skeletal muscles, particularly of the head and neck, resembling opisthotonus or torticollis, may be observed; the eyes may be turned upwards in an oculogyric crisis. Any of these adverse reactions should be reported immediately. Relief may be obtained by the administration of procyclidine (Kemadrin) 5–10 mg (approximate dose) given either by slow intravenous injection or intramuscularly.

(b) *Parkinsonian syndrome*. This unwanted effect of the neuroleptics is said to be more common in the older age group (as is Parkinson's disease). It usually appears after two to three months of treatment. The patient's symptoms resemble those of true parkinsonism: shuffling gait, muscular rigidity, mask-like facies etc.

(c) *Akathisia*. Patients affected by this side-effect are often middle-aged. They are unable to sit or stand still and are continuously on the move, and may complain of feelings of inner restlessness as well. This apparent 'fidgetiness' may also cause the patient to have difficulty in getting to sleep at night. Accurate nursing observations are necessary lest this reaction is misinterpreted as

emotional agitation and treated with further medication. Treatment of akathisia with antiparkinsonian drugs is not usually helpful, but there has been some success with propranolol and benzodiazepines.

(d) Tardive dyskinesia. This serious and potentially irreversible condition is more common in the elderly. It is recognized to be associated with the long-term administration of neuroleptics (but not exclusively), and because a number of patients with this distressing reaction have not responded to treatment, prevention is of the essence. To this end measures which may be taken include so-called 'drug holidays' (temporary withdrawal of medication for perhaps one month in every six); careful and regular drug reviews; discontinuation of drug therapy, at least for a while, at the first hint of symptoms; most importantly, antipsychotic drugs should be prescribed only when absolutely essential and dosage should be as low as possible to obtain relief of the patient's symptoms.

A dominant feature is an excess of involuntary motor activity. Tongue and neck muscles are especially affected; body-rocking movements have been described. Facial symptoms range from occasional movements of the jaw from side to side, and lip and tongue movements which result in mild facial distortions, to those which are incessant and disfiguring.

Hypotensive Effects of Antipsychotic Medication

Postural hypotension is noted particularly with chlorpromazine given intramuscularly. The nurse should ensure the patient does not try to get up too soon afterwards.

Endocrine Disturbance

Some neuroleptics exert hormonal influences such as an increase in prolactin levels in the blood. High levels of this hormone may give rise to menstrual irregularities and milk secretion in non-pregnant women. This can be very upsetting for the patient who may be reassured to some extent when the nurse explains that this is a fairly common and harmless side-effect of medication.

Haematological Effects

Leucopenia, which may lead to fatal agranulocytosis, is fortunately extremely rare, but, because of its acute onset, may be missed on routine blood testing. For this reason it is necessary for the nurse to know the early signs of this reaction, especially when caring for someone receiving chlorpromazine *for the first time* who may be too acutely disturbed and withdrawn to complain of any physical symptoms. A sore throat or a fever may be the first signs. Suspicions may be aroused when the nurse notices the patient holding his throat and grimacing each time he swallows or shivering when the weather is mild.

Skin Reactions

People taking neuroleptics can develop light-sensitive skin reactions. Barrier creams may be of help, but it is preferable to seek shade if outdoors on bright sunny days. Other sensitivity rashes have been noted.

RATIONALE FOR SPECIFIC OBSERVATIONS

Not all patients receiving medication develop adverse effects but should they occur specific observations documented by the nursing staff will facilitate early detection and allow for appropriate intervention (those already discussed in Chapter 7 have been omitted).

Observation	*Rationale*
Patient's blood pressure	Risk of hypotension with antidepressant and neuroleptic drugs
Patient's temperature	Risk of infection due to lowering of white blood count with mianserin, chlorpromazine and clozapine
Patient's weight	Weight gain with antidepressant and neuroleptic drugs
Patient's ability to put out his tongue and keep it out for short period	Inability to stop tongue withdrawing into the mouth may be an early sign of tardive dyskinesia
Sample of handwriting	Quality of subsequent samples will detect evidence of tremor—sign of impending drug-induced parkinsonism with neuroleptic drugs

FURTHER READING

Beeber L (1988) Checking the effects. *Nursing Times* **84**(30): 28–30.

Brooking J, Ritter S & Thomas B (eds) (1992) *Textbook of Pyschiatric and Mental Health Nursing*. Edinburgh: Churchill Livingstone.

Healy D (1993) *Psychiatric Drugs Explained*. London: Mosby.

REFERENCES

Cookson J (1993) Misery blights neuroleptics. *Hospital Doctor* **13**(22): 31.

Cowan P (1988) The physical treatments. In: Rose N (ed.) *Essential Psychiatry*. Oxford: Blackwell Scientific Publications, p 189.

Kay E & Bailie G (1990) Fluoxamine and fluoxetine. *Update* **40**(1): 73–88.

Launer M (1992) Drugs in focus. *Prescribers Journal* **32**(2): 70–73.

Murray J, Walker J & Doyle J (1988) Tyramine in alcohol-free beer. *Lancet* **ii**(8595): 1167–1168.

Priest R (1989) Antidepressants of the future. *British Journal of Psychiatry* **155** (Supplement 6): 7–8.

Reynolds G (1989) Beyond the dopamine hypothesis. The neurochemical pathology of schizophrenia. *British Journal of Psychiatry* **155**: 305–316.

Silverstone T & Turner P (1988) *Drug Treatment in Psychiatry*. London: Routledge and Kegan Paul.

Appendix D
Life Events and Anxiety Rating Scales

LIFE EVENTS SCALE

Life Event	Score
1 Death of spouse	100
2 Divorce	73
3 Marital separation	65
4 Imprisonment	63
5 Death of close family member	63
6 Personal injury or illness	53
7 Marriage	50
8 Fired at work	47
9 Marital reconciliation	45
10 Retirement	45
11 Change in health of family member	44
12 Pregnancy	40
13 Sexual difficulties	39
14 Gain of new family member	39
15 Business readjustment	39
16 Change in financial state	38
17 Death of a close friend	37
18 Change to different line of work	36
19 Change in number of arguments with spouse	35
20 Mortgage over £40 000	31
21 Foreclosure of mortgage or loan	30
22 Change in responsibilities at work	29
23 Son or daughter leaving home	29

24	Trouble with in-laws	29
25	Outstanding personal achievement	28
26	Wife begins or stops work	26
27	Begin or end school	26
28	Change in living conditions	25
29	Revision of personal habits	24
30	Trouble with boss	23
31	Change in work hours or conditions	20
32	Change in residence	20
33	Change in schools	20
34	Change in recreation	19
35	Change in church activities	19
36	Change in social activities	18
37	Mortgage or loan less than £40 000	17
38	Change in sleeping habits	16
39	Change in number of family get-togethers	15
40	Change in eating habits	13
41	Holiday	13
42	Minor violation of the law	11

(Adapted from Holmes TH and Rahe RH (1967) The social readjustments scale. *Journal of Psychosomatic Research*, **11**: 213–218.)

ANXIETY RATING SCALE

SELF RATING OF PROBLEMS

PATIENT .... DATE .... THERAPIST ....

Below are written the agreed definition of your problem or problems. Read through them carefully and initial them.

PROBLEM A ....

.... Patient's signature

PROBLEM B ....

.... Patient's signature

Next you will find two rating scales—a 'feelings scale' and a 'behaviour scale'. For each problem select the number on each scale that best corresponds to the severity of the problem in your case; you may choose 'in between' numbers if this seems appropriate. Write the selected numbers (scores) in the answer boxes alongside the rating scales.

	DATE	/ /	/ /	/ /	/ /	/ /	/ /

FEELINGS SCALE

0	1	2	3	4	5	6	7	8
Never feel at all upset about this problem		Sometimes feel a bit upset about this problem		Often feel quite upset about this problem		Very often feel seriously upset about this problem		Continually feel extremely upset about this problem

A	A	A	A	A	A	A
B	B	B	B	B	B	B

BEHAVIOUR SCALE

0	1	2	3	4	5	6	7	8
Does not interfere with my normal activities		Occasionally interferes with my normal activities		Quite often interferes with my normal activities		Very often interferes with my normal activities		Continually and seriously interferes with my normal activities

A	A	A	A	A	A	A
B	B	B	B	B	B	B

Diary for Keeping Records of Anxiety Rating

HOMEWORK DIARY

WEEK COMMENCING: ....

NAME ....

Goals for the week:
1. ....
2. ....
3. ....
4. ....

0	2	4	6	8
No anxiety	Slight anxiety	Definite anxiety	Marked anxiety	Panic

Session		Goal No.	Task performed	Ratings			Comments: including coping tactics	Co-therapist involvement
Date	Began	Ended			Before	During	End		

Appendix E
Useful Addresses and Telephone Numbers

Every effort has been made to ensure that the following addresses and telephone numbers are current and correct, but the publishers will be most grateful for information regarding any recent changes, along with suggestions for new inclusions in future editions.

Age Concern England
60 Pitcairn Road
Mitcham
Surrey CR4 3LL
Tel: 081–679 8000

Age-Link
Suite 5
The Manor House
The Green
Southall
Middx UB2 4BR
Tel: 071–734 9083

Alcohol Concern
305 Gray's Inn Road
London WC1X 8QF
Tel: 071–833 3471

Alcoholics Anonymous (AA)
General Service Office
PO Box 1
Stonebow House
York YO1 2NJ
Tel: 0904 644026 (admin);
    071–352 3001 (helpline)

Alzheimer's Disease Society
158–160 Balham High Road
London SW12 9BN
Tel: 081–675 6557

Anorexia and Bulimia
    Nervosa Association
Tottenham Women's Health
    Centre
Town Hall Approach
London N15 4RX
Tel: 081–885 3936

Anti-Racist Response and
    Action Group (ARRAG)
c/o 112a The Green
Southall
Middx UB2 4BQ
Tel: 081–574 6019

Association for Post-Natal
    Illness
7 Gowan Avenue
London SW6 6RH
Tel: 071–731 4867

Association for Prevention
of Addiction (APA)
5–7 Tavistock Place
London WC1H 9SS
Tel: 071–383 5071

British Association for
Counselling
37a Sheep Street
Rugby
Warwickshire CV21 3BX
Tel: 0788 78328/9

British Epilepsy Association
Anstey House
40 Hanover Sq
Leeds LS3 1BE
Tel: 0532 439393

British Geriatrics Society
(BGS)
1 St Andrew's Place
Regents Park
London NW1 4LB
Tel: 071–935 4004

Carers National Association
29 Chilworth Mews
London W2 3RG
Tel: 071–724 7776

Help the Aged
16–18 St James's Walk
London EC1R 0BE
Tel: 071–253 0253

Commission for Racial
Equality
Elliott House
10–12 Allington House
London SW1E 5EH
Tel: 071–828 7022

Committee Against Drug
Abuse (CADA)
359 Old Kent Road
London SE1 5JH
Tel: 071–231 1528

Committee on Safety of
Medicines
Market Towers
1 Nine Elms Lane
London SW8 5NQ
Tel: 071–720 2188

Cruse (National
Organization for the
Widowed and their
Children)
Cruse House
126 Sheen Road
Richmond
Surrey TW9 1UR
Tel: 081–940 4818

Depressives Anonymous
(fellowship of)
36 Chestnut Avenue
Beverley
North Humberside HU17
9QU
Tel: 0482 860619

Families Anonymous (FA)
310 Finchley Road
London NW3 7AG
Tel: 071–731 8060

Gamblers Anonymous and
Gam-Anon
PO Box 88
London SW10 0CU
Tel: 071–352 3060

King's Fund Centre (KFC)
126 Albert Street
London NW1 7NF
Tel: 071-267 6111

Medical Council on
    Alcoholism (MCA)
1 St Andrew's Place
London NW1 4LB
Tel: 071-487 4445

Mental After Care
    Association
Bainbridge House
Bainbridge Street
London WC1A 1HP
Tel: 071-436 6194

MIND (National Association
    for Mental Health)
22 Harley Street
London W1N 2ED
Tel: 071-637 0741

Narcotics Anonymous
PO Box 417
London SW10 0DP
Tel: 071-351 6794

National Association of
    Citizens' Advice Bureaux
115-123 Pentonville Road
London N1 9LZ
Tel: 071-833 2181

National Schizophrenia
    Fellowship
28 Castle Street
Kingston-upon-Thames KT1
    1SS
Tel: 081-547 3937

National Society for Epilepsy
Chalfont Centre for Epilepsy
Chalfont St Peter
Gerrards Cross
Bucks SL9 0RJ
Tel: 02407 3991

Phobic Action
Greater London House
547-551 High Road
London E11 4PR
Tel: 081-558 6012

Phobics Society
4 Cheltenham Road
Chorlton-cum-Hardy
Manchester M21 1QN
Tel: 061-881 1937

Samaritans
17 Uxbridge Road
Slough
Berkshire SL1 1SN
Tel: 0753 32713

SANE (Schizophrenia—a
    National Emergency)
5th Floor
120 Regent Street
London W1A 5FE
Tel: 071-494 4840

Schizophrenia Association of
    Great Britain (SAGB)
Bryn Hyfryd, The Crescent
Bangor
Gwynedd LL57 2AG
Tel: 0248 354048

Scottish Council on Alcohol,
    The
137-145 Sauchiehall Street
Glasgow G2 3EW
Tel: 041-333 9677

Society for Advancement
of Research into Anorexia
(SARA)
Stanthorpe
New Pound
Wisborough Green
West Sussex RH14 0EJ
Tel: 0403 700210

Standing Conference of
Ethnic Minority Senior
Citizens
Ethnic Minority Resource
Centre
5–5a Westminster Bridge
Road
London SW1 7XW
Tel: 071–928 0095

Standing Conference on
Drug Abuse (SCODA)
1–4 Hatton Place
Hatton Garden
London EC1N 8ND
Tel: 071–430 2341

Stress Syndrome Foundation
Cedar House
Yalding
Kent ME18 6JD

Tavistock Institute of Human
Relations
Tavistock Centre
Belsize Lane
London NW3 5BA
Tel: 071–435 7111 ext 2383

Terence Higgins Trust
52–54 Gray's Inn Road
London WC1X 8JU
Tel: 071–242 1010

Index

BRISTOL CITY COUNCIL
LIBRARY SERVICE

BRISTOL
REFERENCE LIBRARY

COLLEGE GREEN

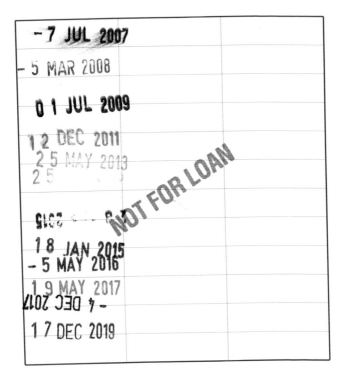